NUTRITION
CANCER AND YOU

What you need to know,
and where to start

NUTRITION
CANCER AND YOU

What you need to know,
and where to start

by

Susan Calhoun
and Jane Bradley

Addax Publishing Group
Lenexa, Kansas

Addax Publishing Group
8643 Hauser Drive · Suite 235
Lenexa, Kansas 66215
913-438-5333 · 800-598-5550

Edited by Michael McKenzie

Printed in the United States of America
96 97 98 99 00 01   10 9 8 7 6 5 4 3 2 1

Library of Congress Catalog Card Number: 96-85765

ISBN: 1-886110-06-9

Endorsements

This book has been a helpful resource to many participants at the Bloch Cancer Support Center. It was one of the first books to be acquired by our library and is seldom checked in.
— TRISH MILLER, Former Director
R.A. Bloch Cancer Support Center

As an oncology nurse for the past 10 years, I have always known the importance of nutrition for the oncology patient. These authors have given this topic high priority, as well as a thorough overview of nutrition. The content is precise enough for nursing use, yet written in a format that can be understood by anyone. As a nurse and patient advocate, I would recommend this as reading for every oncology nurse, patient, and/or family member. — PAULA BOMAR, R.N. OCN

Very informative for patients with limited nutritional knowledge.
— DANA LEWIS, R.N. OCN

Gives cancer patients the nutritional basics they need to be able to maintain/improve their nutritional status.
— MELANIE SIMPSON, R.N. OCN

The authors took every precaution to assure that the information in this book is in accordance with current recommendations and practices. However, ongoing research and a constant flow of information about cancer can change practices.

Our objective and passion is to help the patient and caregivers communicate easier with a physician about concerns over the patient's unique nutritional needs. No part of this book is intended to replace the instructions or advice of the physician.

We urge you to consult a physician on all matters relating to health.

Contents

Foreword

Host factors such as functional level and weight loss have long been known to have a significant impact on clinical outcomes for cancer patients. As early as 1932 research pointed out that malnutrition was a major factor contributing to mortality.

Since then, research offers a greater understanding of the changes in metabolic pathways leading to cancer cachexia (severe malnutrition and muscle wasting). Now scientists aim their research at uncovering the underlying mechanisms, such as production of so-called cytokines or humoral factors. These are chemicals, made either directly by the cancer or as a response by the patient's body to the cancer, which have many effects on the body's handling of food and calories, as well as appetite.

Some experimental evidence suggests that blocking or eliminating these factors will help reverse the cachectic state. This raises the hope of future intervention aimed at the root cause of cancer cachexia.

Another approach to malnutrition is through successful treatment of the cancer itself. This is known to reverse tumor cachexia. This has long been the focus of the medical profession, and we have seen much progress in many types of cancer treatment. As the authors pointed out, aggressive support is increasingly important to allow patients to complete aggressive treatment plans. Physicians and patients must understand that to maximize the benefit of the treatment, the cachexia must be addressed as part of the overall approach, and not as an afterthought.

Until we become more effective at these approaches, intervention at malnutrition is aimed at "keeping up." Several devices allow delivery of calories and nutrients with a specific type of each tailored to the individual patient.

Decisions regarding this are best made in an interactive way by the physician, nutritional team and patient. The basic knowledge contained in this book will remove some of the stigma of being "fed through a tube" and promote wider use of nutritional support.

One of the primary themes is that wider use will come through a greater awareness of the importance of nutritional support, both by providers and patients. Several factors lend themselves to this greater awareness: an increasing emphasis on the quality of life, the team approach in which other professions, including nutritionists, are involved more often and more quickly, and a shift from a paternalistic medical profession to a more interactive model in which patients play an active role in decision making.

To play this role, patients will need the information this book provides in such clear, basic, practical terms.

— SCOTT C. COZAD, M.D.
Medical Director
Parvin Road Radiation Oncology

Introduction

Any belief that nutrition and vitamins alone can cure cancer is misplaced. They can help a great deal, though, if you have some basic knowledge about healthful eating. This guide will assist you.

One of our strongest purposes is to arm you with proper information with which to communicate nutritional concerns to the physician, nurse, dietician or other providers of care for a cancer patient, whether it's you or your loved one.

Good nutrition is not therapy, in and of itself. However, research definitely supports the notion that good nutrition provides a *vital link in the treatment plan for cancer patients.*

Simply eating all your vegetables might not be enough. You must know the importance and sources of calories found in protein, carbohydrates and fat, along with the important vitamins and minerals.

Using our more than 25 years of combined experience in the nutrition field, we let one main purpose guide us through this book—to inform you about certain foods and eating habits so you can work with care providers during treatment to maintain proper nourishment that can be supportive.

We have outlined specific ways to add *motivation, good sense and good taste* to the eating habits of the cancer patient. You'll enjoy the special recipes, charts, tips and questions as aides.

Nutrition is a relatively new science. Its impact still is not fully understood in our rapidly-advancing scientific and technological world. Research is mounting, yet remains inconclusive, and opinions about nutrition vacillate. However, apart from any ongoing debates, our experience and studies support two universal premises regarding nutrition:

- It can be very supportive in the treatment of cancer

- It can, in some cases, sustain the patient

Through our practical experience and by thoroughly reviewing research, we know this: By maintaining a well-nourished body, you increase the probability of:

- Handling the stress of cancer

- Reducing side effects

- Increase tolerance for more "therapeutically appropriate" doses of chemotherapy and radiation

- Most significantly, *improving the quality of your life*

We have worked in several roles in the field of nutrition. We helped develop Nutritional Support Teams in hospitals, and we have provided continuing education programs to professionals, such as physicians, pharmacists, dieticians and nurses.

We also stay abreast of the studies and works of *The American Society for Parenteral and Enteral Nutrition,* a professional organization dedicated to nutritional research.

The information from this research is designed to help you understand and implement the unique nutritional plan for the patient's body during treatment for cancer.

— JANE AND SUSAN

CHAPTER 1

Why Eating Well Is Important

Proper nourishment helps you feel better, and helps fight the effects of cancer and your treatments. Nutrition is important to your recovery. No special diet by itself will replace the proven methods of treatment. However, a nutritionally-balanced diet is essential during treatment time so your body can best fight the disease.

- Scientific studies reveal that cancer patients have a better chance of a good recovery from surgery, chemotherapy and radiation if nutrition improves before, during and after the treatments.

- By keeping your body's system strong you increase your chances of a favorable response to therapy.

- Good eating habits make the patient less suscep- tible to infections that could weaken the body and cause timely treatments to be delayed.

■ Cancer patients who eat a balance of protein, fat, and carbohydrates are better able to maintain strength.

■ Adequate calories minimize the breakdown of muscle, which the body needs for energy, and enhances the repair of tissues.

■ When you eat less your body breaks down its own storage of fat and muscle that provide needed nutrients. Fat surrounding the organs protects them; it is more susceptible to break down than fat in the larger storage sites like the thigh or stomach. Recognizing this and addressing it early on with planned nutrition — before deficits occur — can minimize losses.

Providing nutritional care for a patient with cancer is difficult. Often he or she is not hungry because of the illness and/or treatment — just at the time that nutritional requirements rise far above normal.

Medical experts don't understand all the reasons for weight loss during cancer therapy. We know it often goes beyond simply taking in fewer calories. Many changes in the body's system pose special challenges to meeting nutritional needs adequately.

Even without complications or nutritional deficits, cancer alters metabolism. Therefore a patient's needs change, too.

Cancer increases normal metabolism (in approximately 60 percent of patients), thus calories burn quicker. Recognition and identification of these changes will help you respond to them and offset their effects.

Initial changes in metabolism often are subtle. Be forewarned: *Malnutrition can set in before any visible loss in weight occurs.* At first the signs and effects of malnutrition might go unnoticed, because the symptoms can be as silent as, for example, high blood pressure. Significant damage can occur before the symptoms surface.

Low protein intake compromises the immune functions long before someone outwardly looks malnourished. You can see why it is so important to become fully educated on how best to offset any deficiencies before they exact a toll.

You have a far easier challenge to maintain reasonably good nutrition as a precaution against vital depletion than to try to revitalize someone who is already debilitated.

At every turn, we readily see the immense value of eating well.

CHAPTER 2

General Advice For Eating Well

In the circumstances Chapter 1 foretold — if a patient has lost appetite; taste buds are altered, digestion is off track, and fortitude has weakened — the rules change.

You must adapt nutritional guidelines. The primary goal: *Get the most nutrition from the least amount of effort.* With that in mind, use these hints to minimize problems for both the patient and the caregiver in establishing a balanced diet.

Environment

- Vary the colors of food to make it look more pleasing. Use reds, yellows and greens to advantage.

- Soft background music, fresh-cut flowers and colorful place settings make mealtime more enjoyable.

- Use good china, silverware and tablecloth . . . table decor traditionally reserved for holidays or special occasions.

- Have meals with family and friends, not in isolation (especially not in a bedroom, whenever it can be avoided).

- Associate meal times with pleasant feelings to help the patient want to eat more.

- Eye appeal and aura make a great deal of difference. Never underestimate ambience.

Using "up" days

Take advantage of "feel-good" days to eat meals that have more nutritional momentum; the body thereby stores nutrients for later use. When energy levels are higher, the patient can prepare extra nutritionally-dense meals to freeze for later use when he or she is not up to cooking.

Living Alone

If the patient lives alone, meal preparation can be difficult, especially because of fatigue. Make arrangements for the service "Meals on Wheels." Ask your doctor, nurse, dietitian, or the American Cancer Society about the availability in your community. Many churches provide meal delivery.

Keep cupboards stocked

Stock the cupboards with foods that are convenient to prepare, yet nutritious. Some manufacturers make fortified soups, cereals, milk shakes, puddings, such as Ensure, Carnation Instant Breakfast or Sustacal. These usually require simply mixing with hot water or milk. Such products are highly concentrated in protein and calories.

Work with a team of professionals

Before trying different remedies that you read about or that friends suggest (such as low fat/high protein diets, juice fasting, herbal cleansing), be sure that symptoms are not of a nature calling for medical attention. Even if you think your questions or concerns are minor, immediately discuss them with your doctor and other care providers.

Vitamin supplements

Always check with your doctor before taking any vitamin or mineral supplement. Loss of taste can result from a zinc deficiency. Because this nutrient is easily depleted by prolonged or extreme stress, a zinc supplement might help. But, talk to your doctor first, as lab tests may be in order.

Use precaution in using manufactured herbs. Many concentrated herbs in capsule form are less regulated by governing agencies, hence you can't be assured of the quality. The crops that produced them might have been treated with toxic chemicals to enhance mass production. Especially herbs from other countries, where standards and regulations are suspect.

Some herbs are very potent, and some contain naturally-occurring aldehydes that tax the liver excessively. Some herbs have high levels of naturally-occurring hormones, such as estrogen, possibly undesirable in a cancer condition.

Until a clearer picture appears in the regulation and application of herbs, you are prudent to remain conservative and to get your nutrients from whole foods and fresh herbs from the garden (parsley, chives, mint, etc.) for flavor enhancement.

Avoid raw and rare

Bacteria tends to gather in uncooked or undercooked eggs, meat and fish. This is no time to add such stress on a cancer patient's body, making it deal with the risk of food poisoning or infection. A low white blood count during treatment could compromise the patient's ability to fight infection.

Here's an example of how innocence can beg trouble. Eggnog is a good source of calories and protein, but it also may be a source of trouble because the egg content might be contaminated. Be safe: used cooked egg recipes only. Meanwhile, for a fun treat, try "Mock Eggnog" (found in the recipe section).

Also, the Federal Drug Administration recommends that persons with cancer avoid raw or undercooked shellfish, especially mollusks (oysters, clams, mussels and scallops). They can cause serious problems. So be certain that the fish are thoroughly cooked.

Tips for increasing calories and protein

- Use nut butters on vegetable sticks and crackers
- Add butter or margarine to soups, vegetables, pastas, breads
- Add grated cheese to vegetables, casseroles, salads
- Use cream instead of milk in soups, cereals, coffee
- Use mayonnaise on sandwiches
- Use ample gravies and sauces over foods
- Use milk instead of water to reconstitute canned soups
- Keep chewy granola bars on hand
- Keep pretzels, nuts, raisins, and hard candy available for snacks
- Add brown sugar, honey, or syrups to hot cereals and pancakes
- Drop a scoop of sherbet into a tall glass of ginger ale
- Add dry milk to soups, casseroles, hot cereal, and baked products
- Lace hot cereals and bran muffins with blackstrap molasses, which is rich in B vitamins, iron and calcium

- Spread cream cheese or peanut butter on rice cakes

- Grind up sunflower, pumpkin or sesame seeds into cereals or baked goods

- And, for something different, use tofu in casseroles, soups and stir-fry dishes. It is bland, therefore it blends with the taste of the prepared dish, and it is packed with protein and calcium.

Minimize time in food preparation

Saving time and energy is important so that the body gets its needed rest. Sometimes nutrition gets compromised because the patient is too tired to prepare meals.

- Arrange for others to cook whenever possible

- Look into "Meals on Wheels"

- Eat out when the patient feels up to it; otherwise, take advantage of restaurant take-out or delivery services.

- Whenever "down time" for surgery or treatments occurs, have a helpers list to keep caregivers in tune with the patient's needs

- Keep a general grocery list, and write out menus of meals that family members can prepare easily

- Make use of disposable dishes, napkins, pans when help is not available

- Take advantage of mixes and frozen foods, leaving more leisure and family time

- When the patient is too tired to eat, go for protein. Small sips of a canned protein shake, for instance, might provide an energy lift so he or she will feel like eating later.

CHAPTER 3

Minimizing Eating Problems

Nutritional effects from cancer treatment range from mild, intermittent disturbances to problems that can become severe, even permanent. So how do you maintain a patient's optimum nutritional status? How can you overcome some of the side effects of cancer and its therapies? Let's take a look at the various symptoms and note how each can be approached.

Some side effects of cancer and treatments

- Taste changes and loss of appetite
- Feelings of fullness
- Nausea and vomiting
- Diarrhea and cramps
- Lactose intolerance
- Constipation
- Mouth and throat problems
- Bloating and heartburn
- Excessive weight gain and fluid retention

Taste changes and loss of appetite

A patient can lose taste and appetite many ways — naturally, or induced by sources of treatment. Cancer itself sometimes produces substances that affect the part of the brain that triggers hunger. Appetite also can be affected by alterations in the taste of food.

Taste changes can result from radiation therapy, especially to the head and neck region. Damage to healthy tissues sometimes occurs. The extent of irritation or damage depends on the type of radiation therapy, the area irradiated, the dose, and the size of the tumor.

Radiation to the head and neck also can cause decreased saliva and mouth "blindness," which might set in two weeks after treatment begins and last from several months to one year after treatment ends. The loss of saliva decreases the ability to taste foods. Further, damage to the microvilli of the taste cells suppress the normal taste sensations.

Oncology medications can cause changes in taste, too. Foods that you previously liked might seem too sweet or sour, bitter or metallic. Whenever these taste changes occur, it is very important to find alternative ways to overcome them while still providing the body with adequate amounts of protein and calories.

Protein is essential because of its effect on building and maintaining the immune system. Red meat is typically a rich source for protein, yet red meat might have a bitter taste. Minimize the bitterness by marinating the meat in soy sauce or sweet wine, or by serving the previously cooked meat at a chilled temperature. If bitterness remains, substitute chicken or fish for the red-meat protein.

Zinc deficiency sometimes creates taste alterations in a cancer patient. Diet deficiency doesn't necessarily cause this; researchers believe the tumor takes zinc out of the system. Additionally, many drug therapies display a tendency to deplete zinc levels.

Discuss the ramifications with a physician before starting zinc supplements. Zinc that reaches high levels can precipitate copper and possibly cause a mineral imbalance. Your doctor or dietitian will recommend needed dosages.

Protein requirements rise in cancer patients during periods of metabolic stress to the body. Demands can range from 1.0 to 1.5 grams or more for each kilogram of body weight.

To determine daily protein requirements, convert your weight to kilograms (divide your weight in pounds by 2.2) and multiply by 1.0 to 1.5 to ascertain the range or total grams of protein required daily.

Protein Guideline Formula for a 150-pound male

150 divided by 2.2 = 68.18 kilograms

68 kilograms x 1.5 = 102 grams protein/day

Before starting a plan, talk to a doctor or dietitian for specific numbers and recommendations, because needs vary from case to case. Kidney failure (renal) patients, for example, must restrict protein intake. The protein formula simply provides a guideline.

When attention to protein demands becomes an oversight, the patient may be at risk for malnutrition, and playing "catch up" is difficult.

PROTEIN FOOD CHART

- Beef or other red meat
- Poultry
- Fish
- Cheese
- Eggs
- Tofu
- Lentils

- Dried peas
- Dried beans
- Tuna
- Milk shakes
- Custards
- Egg salad
- Yogurt

Feelings of fullness

When the patient feels full, resort to foods high in carbohydrates, such as toast, gelatin, and juices. They digest quicker than fatty or fried foods.

Go for smaller, more frequent meals, and plan for liquids after consumption. It is more important to concentrate on the nutritional content of each meal than the number of meals or the amount of food eaten.

Nausea and vomiting

These two common side effects raise danger signals because, if prolonged, they can lead to imbalances in fluid and electrolytes. A physician may prescribe antinausea medication to help. Nausea might be caused by abdominal or pelvic radiation, resulting in altered function of the intestines.

Research reveals multiple causes of nausea, such as medication. If vomiting persists more than 24 hours contact a physician.

An electrolyte replacement drink might become necessary to replenish losses such as sodium and potassium. These specialty drinks quickly rebalance the system.

Helpful hints for nausea and vomiting

- Eat frequent small meals ■ Avoid strong odors
- Eat cool or room temperature foods
- Increase fluid intake ■ Limit high fat food intake
- Avoid spicy foods
- Use sweet carbonated beverages to help nausea
- Eat salty foods rather than sweet ones
- Coca-Cola syrup is an old fashioned remedy for nausea (if you can fint it)
- "Emetrol" is available without a prescription

Foods to help with nausea

- Crackers and toast
- Sherbert
- Popsicles
- Tart foods
- Pretzels

Diarrhea and Cramps

Malabsorption, a condition created when the intestines incur damage during radiation therapy, is one of the many causes of diarrhea. Radiation destroys cells that normally produce the fluids necessary to digest certain food components — fat, protein, carbohydrates and other nutrients.

Malabsorption requires a special "predigested" diet to resolve the diarrhea. If malabsorption evolves, a dietitian will be helpful in outlining dietary recommendations.

Diarrhea also results from certain colon surgeries, but this type of diarrhea usually clears up shortly after surgery, and large electrolyte losses are limited. Diarrhea caused from chemotherapy is usually of short duration, also, due to the rapid recovery of the gastrointestinal tract.

Cramping might take place after the intake of certain foods that cause gas, including:

- Cabbage
- Onions
- Beans
- Garlic
- High fiber foods (broccoli, corn, cauliflower)
- High lactose foods (milk and other dairy products)

If diarrhea sets in, avoid:

- Greasy, fatty, or fried food
- Alcohol
- Caffeine

Diarrhea can deplete the body of potassium. For potassium replacement, eat:

- Potatoes (especially the skins)
- Apricots
- Lemon juice

- Peaches
- Honeydew melon

If diarrhea persists more than 24 hours or contains blood, notify a physician.

Lactose intolerance

Some patients experience diarrhea because of an intolerance to milk and diary products. As we grow older we gradually reduce our tolerance to lactose, a milk sugar that is broken down by the enzyme lactase. With insufficient lactase, the body won't digest milk sugar.

Problems associated with insufficient lactase usually occur more rapidly after the administering of chemotherapy, radiation to abdominal area, antibiotics, or any treatment that affects the gastrointestinal tract. Typically, the symptoms of cramping, gas and diarrhea disappear after the treatment stops, or when the intestine has had ample time to heal. However, sometimes the problem recurs and requires long-term change in eating habits.

Generally a doctor will recommend a diet low in lactose. Some people who are lactose intolerant manage well with buttermilk and yogurt because they have been altered in processing. If milk becomes a problem, many soy milks on the market have improved tastes, especially if served very cold.

Health food stores usually have a large variety of milk-substitute products to choose from. Because caloric requirements are high, choose the soy milk with full fat rather than the low-fat selections.

Reducing lactose-containing foods from a diet requires careful reading of labels. Foods with lactose can include breads cooked with milk, all cheeses except naturally aged, ice cream, cream, custards, cream fillings, gravies with milk, and any prepared products that contain dry milk solids.

In the dairy case at many grocery stores you'll find tablets that supply the enzyme lactase to help in the digestion of milk sugars. Add the tablet to milk 24 hours before use, rendering the milk more easily digested, yet without compromising the nutritional value of the milk.

Lactose-containing foods

- Milk (liquid or dry)
- Ice cream
- Cream (sour and sweet)
- Cheese (exception: naturally aged cheeses)
- Desserts with cream filling
- Bread and cereal items containing milk
- Powdered coffee creamer
- Creamed vegetables and meat
- Creamed soups
- Sauces
- Party dips
- Instant potatoes

Constipation

Certain cancer-fighting drugs, chemotherapy, pain medications, diet lacking sufficient fiber and fluid, intestinal spasms, infrequent exercise, and stress all are known to contribute to constipation.

Tips for minimizing constipation:

- Exercise; even moderate amounts help
- Increase fluid in diet; drink 6–8 glasses of water daily
- Increase fiber; include more whole grains, breads, bran muffins, vegetables, raw fruits, raisins, apricots, prunes, and nuts
- Take natural laxatives, such as warm prune juice with lemon added
- If constipation persists, talk to a doctor about stool softeners or artificial bulk products. Avoid taking laxatives without a doctor's advice.

Mouth and throat problems

A dry or sore mouth from radiation or chemotherapy makes eating extremely difficult, and certainly undesirable. Mouth sores, tender gums, and inflammation of the throat foster irritation and make swallowing difficult at best. The patient's interest in eating reaches all-time lows when pain is the reward.

While some foods increase discomfort, careful selection of foods to counteract the food tract problems can sometimes help the patient feel better about attempting to eat.

For dry mouth:

- Rinse mouth often with saline solution
- Drink plenty of fluid
- Suck on crushed ice
- Suck on hard candy to stimulate saliva
- Ask a doctor to prescribe an artificial saliva product
- Take a sip of fluid with each bite of food
- Make foods moist by adding sauces, gravies, melted butter, salad dressing, broth, sour cream or mayonnaise

- Dip biscuits and crackers in tea or coffee
- Cook food until it's soft before blending it
- Apply a lanolin-based moisturizer to cracked or chapped lips every 2-4 hours
- Use a room humidifier

For sore mouth and throat:

- Avoid hot foods; cooler foods are more comfortable to eat
- Try bananas, peaches, milk shakes, cottage cheese, apricots, watermelon
- Avoid highly-acidic foods (tomato sauce, orange and grapefriut juice)
- Cut food into small pieces
- Mash, blend, or puree foods
- Try baby foods
- Avoid foods that scratch and irritate the mouth lining
- Avoid alcohol
- Avoid tobacco and smoking
- Ask physician to prescribe medicine that numbs mouth sores
- Use lozenges or sprays
- An occupational therapist knows resources to help with swallowing if this problem is persistent.

The following foods can help alleviate symptoms associated with an uncomfortable mouth or throat.

- Milkshakes, malt
- Creamed or pureed soups
- Whipped potatoes
- Pastas with cheese sauce
- Rice
- Ground meat
- Soft-cooked eggs, coddled or soft-scrambled
- Soft french toast (try with melted butter and cinnamon sugar on top)
- Pancakes with syrup
- Mashed bananas sprinkled with nutmeg
- Non-citric juices—pear, apricot, apple
- Tofu mixed into soft casseroles
- Sweetened tea
- Yogurt, sour cream, cottage cheese
- Ice cream, sherbet, fudgesicles, popsicles
- Pudding and custard
- High-calorie, high-protein liquid supplements.

Bloating

Some foods contribute to the production of gas in the stomach or intestines. Sometimes nervousness causes a person to swallow too much air while eating. Malabsorption problems from radiation to the stomach can cause incomplete digestion of food, thereby causing gas. Sometimes bloating or distention are attributable to lack of exercise.

To alleviate bloating problems:

- Low-fat foods that digest more easily
- Eat slowly
- Avoid gas-producing foods such as beans, garlic, onions, cabbage
- Increase exercise
- Stop eating when discomfort sets in
- Use gas-reducing medicine recommended by a doctor

Weight and fluid retention

Weight gain can be a side effect of treatment, of medication (especially cortisone derivatives and hormones), and of malnutrition. Such weight gain is generally water retention.

Although weight gain typically results from treatments, protein malnutrition also causes it. This is different from protein-calorie malnutrition, which profoundly wastes lean muscle tissue ("marasmus").

With absolute protein malnutrition ("kwashiorkor"), profuse internal depletion takes place, yet on the surface the person still would look nourished because they might be receiving enough calories from fat and carbohydrate sources.

Protein malnutrition creates a bloated appearance, much the same as the look in photographs of Third World children with distended bellies. You will read more description of this phenomenon in Chapter 5, *Basics of Nutrition*.

If a patient appears to gain weight, bring it to a doctor's attention so he can determine the cause and make recommendations. He might suggest a reduction in salt in the diet, or a diuretic. If protein malnutrition is the cause, lab tests can measure to what degree.

Regardless of the cause, this is no time to go on a weight-loss diet. The body needs nutrients for maintenance and repair right now, and this must remain a high priority.

A patient gaining weight may want to reduce salt intake, high-fat foods, and replenish with high-quality protein foods.

Heartburn

Certain foods and medicines make a person more susceptible to heartburn by increasing the acid in the stomach.

Avoid:

- Very spicy foods
- Fried and greasy foods
- Alcohol
- Coffee

Eat smaller meals more often so food passes through the stomach more quickly. If heartburn continues, speak to a doctor about antacids and a schedule for using them.

While all suggestions presume to improve a patient's comfort and nutrition, he or she will have to experiment to discover what works. All the points highlighted in this chapter are common, but they don't cover the entire gamut of effects from all forms of cancer and treatments. Therefore, please discuss every concern you have with a team of care providers, especially if a particular problem doesn't subside within a reasonable time.

CHAPTER 4

Eating But Still Losing Weight?

Despite the very best efforts to keep well-nourished by eating well, at times it is still not enough to maintain ideal weight. Meeting nutritional needs is much more demanding during illness and treatment and a simple, balanced diet sometimes rates inadequately as the sole source of your nutrition.

Fortunately, many alternatives exist when your food intake isn't enough. The four main ones to consider in meeting your nutritional goals are:

1. Oral diet

2. Liquid meal replacements

3. Enteral nutrition (tube feedings)

4. Parenteral nutrition (intravenous feedings)

These four methods can be used individually or in conjunction with one another, short- or long-term. Specialty products and regimens help tailor the methods to specific needs.

41

Balanced Oral Diet

A balanced diet provides the body with adequate protein, calories, vitamins and minerals to meet the high demands created by the cancer. Increase the likelihood of a patient having well-balanced meals by planning ahead and making diet menus. Monitor meals with a checklist to ensure reaching necessary goals. A doctor might involve a dietitian to make recommendations and instruction in keeping a food diary. Follow these food groups and suggested serving sizes for assistance:

Enriched grain products

This food group is plentiful in B vitamins that help with digestion. They are a good source of carbohydrates to give energy and are rich in iron for building the blood. Whole grain products are also a good source of other vitamins and minerals.

You should include 6–11 servings every day. Some grain products include:

- Cereal (whole grains)
- Breads (whole grains such as wheat or rye)
- Pastas
- Rice
- Beans
- Crackers
- Pancakes, waffles, crepes

Fruits and vegetables

Fruits and vegetables are an excellent source of Vitamin A which helps maintain mucous membranes during radiation therapy. They also contain vitamin C to aid in the body's defense against infection. Eat 2–4 servings of fruit every day and include one from a citrus juice. Eat 3–5 servings every day of vegetables.

Fruits

- Citrus (lemons, oranges, grapefruit)
- Melons
- Strawberries
- Pineapple
- Apricots
- Peaches
- Bananas

Vegetables

- Potatoes
- Squash
- Spinach
- Peas
- Cabbage
- Lettuce
- Tomatos
- Green beans
- Broccoli
- Yams

Dairy products

These products will provide needed calcium and vitamins A,B, and D. The calcium and vitamin D are especially important for your bones and teeth. The B vitamins will help your nervous system and will be good for the skin and hair. Vitamin A bolsters the immune system. You should have 2–3 servings from the dairy group each day. The items below are also good sources of protein.

Milk: Make a mixture of fortified milk by mixing ⅓ cup of dry milk powder to 8 ounces of milk. Use this mixture of fortified milk for gravies and sauces. Use half and half instead of evaporated milk in soups and puddings. Cook cereals in milk instead of water.

Cheeses: Add to casseroles, desserts and baked goods. Use cream cheese and margarine on bread and rolls or serve cheese with fresh fruit.

Food

A Guide

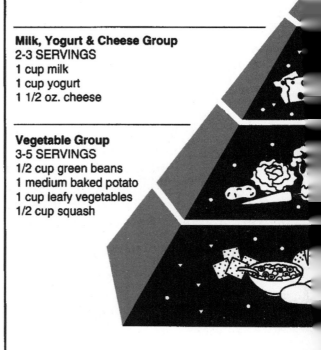

Fats, Oils & Sweets
USE SPARINGLY

Milk, Yogurt & Cheese Group
2-3 SERVINGS
1 cup milk
1 cup yogurt
1 1/2 oz. cheese

Vegetable Group
3-5 SERVINGS
1/2 cup green beans
1 medium baked potato
1 cup leafy vegetables
1/2 cup squash

Source: U.S. Department of Agriculture and U.S. Departmen

'amid
Choices

KEY
⬜ Fat (naturally occurring and added)
🔻 Sugars (added)
These symbols show fats, oils and added sugars in foods.

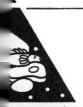

Meat, Poultry, Fish, Dry Beans,
Eggs & Nuts Group
2-3 SERVINGS
2-3 oz. lean meat, fish or poultry
1 egg
1/2 cup cooked dry peas or beans

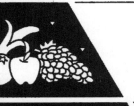

Fruit Group
2-4 SERVINGS
1 banana
1 medium pear
1/2 cup diced fruit
3/4 cup juice

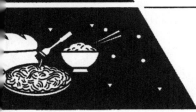

Bread, Cereal, Rice
& Pasta Group
6-11 SERVINGS
1/2 cup pasta
1 slice bread
1 whole-grain dinner roll
1 oz. whole-grain crackers
1 oz. cereal, such as Whole Grain Total

Human Services

Meats or meat alternatives
Daily requirements for this group are 2–3 servings per day. These foods may include:

- Poultry
- Fish
- Beef
- Pork
- Lamb
- Dried peas or beans
- Soy burgers

Increasing your protein and calories
High-calorie, high protein foods are most efficient in providing enough nutrients for your body. Here are some ways you could increase the caloric content of your food:

- Peanut butter on crackers or toast
- Honey as a sweetener in coffee, tea, and cereals
- Mayonnaise on sandwiches and in casseroles
- Cream cheese in casseroles and in cheesecake
- Glucose polymers, in liquids, sauces, gravies, and casseroles. (These often can be found in health food stores marketed as sports drinks.)
- Whipped cream on puddings, gelatin, and desserts

Good sources of protein
Below is a listing of some of foods with high to moderate levels of protein.

Meats
- Hamburger
- Roast beef
- Baked ham
- Turkey and chicken
- T-bone steak
- Meatloaf
- Baked fish

Cereals and grains

- Cream of wheat
- Oatmeal
- Macaroni

Dairy products

- Milk
- Yogurt
- Buttermilk
- Ice cream
- Cheese
- Puddings

Soups

- Lentil soup
- Navy bean soup
- Cream of Broccoli
- Split pea soup
- Cream of Mushroom

Nutrients from a normal oral diet are best if you are able to meet all of your calorie and protein demands. Remember your requirements may be increased at this time due to the metabolic stress of the cancer. We will discuss in a later chapter how to assess your nutritional needs and how to monitor them to make sure you stay in the optimum range. If meeting these demands becomes difficult it is extremely important that you move to a more aggressive method to supply your body's needs. The next step is supplementing your diet with products known as "nutritional supplements."

Nutritional supplements

Nutritional supplements fall into two groups: "nourishments" and "medical nutritionals."

Nourishments are products that are meant to be used to supplement your regular diet. They are fortified with increased amounts of calories and protein. These may be liquid drinks or can be fortified soups, puddings, bars, etc. These products are not meant to be a sole source of nutrition long term but are fine as an adjunct to a regular diet. These products may include sport shakes or power bars.

"Medical nutritionals" differ from nourishment in that they are complete meal replacements and can provide total balanced nutrition for an extended period. Medical nutritionals may be used either as sole source of nutrition or may also supplement your regular diet. Medical nutritionals are generally lactose free to eliminate lactose intolerance problems, gluten free for individuals with allergies to wheat, and usually offer a form containing liquid fiber to aid in bowel functioning. Two examples of medical nutritionals are Ensure or Sustacal.

Both nourishments and medical nutritionals may be purchased in a supermarket or drug store. Your dietitian or physician can give you information on which type and formulation would best fit your needs.

Evaluating nutritional supplements

A good supplement should provide 9–12 grams of protein and 225–355 calories in an 8 ounce serving. A variety of supplements are available including a high calorie formula, high protein formula, or a fiber containing formula. Make sure that you compare prices and read labels carefully. Some supplements may contain only half of the amount of protein, yet may be the same price as a high-protein supplement. In a recent price comparison a difference of $2–$3 dollars per 6-pack difference was noticed depending upon the store. Improved flavors and a large variety of flavors helps make these products very palatable and helps improve patient compliance.

Unflavored nutritional supplements are also available for patients suffering taste alterations. Many times a regular supplement will taste too sweet and a more bland flavor is sought. These unflavored products can also be mixed with the flavored supplements to bring the degree of sweetness to the desired point. These unflavored supplements are typically used for tube feedings when flavor is not an issue and are not as accessible through the retail market but may be ordered by any pharmacy. Ask your dietitian or physician for more specific information on which would be best for you.

Specialty products are also available. For patients with diabetes a special formulation can be used with a blend specifically for glucose intolerant patients to keep blood sugars from rising due to the feeding product.

Supplements are an excellent way of adding to your regular diet or for providing a total source of nutrition if you are unable to eat any regular food at all. If swallowing is difficult or other problems continue to persist and weight loss occurs the next aggressive step in the continuum of support must be considered.

Enteral feedings

To this point, we have discussed two types of feedings: *regular diet* and *nutritional supplements.*

A third type of feeding is "enteral nutrition." Enteral feedings are also called tube feedings due to the way the nourishment is delivered to the patient. With this type of feeding, nutrients are delivered through a tube that bypasses the mouth and taste buds, and liquid nutrition is fed directly into the digestive system.

Enteral feedings not new

Tube feedings have actually been used for a long time dating back as far as several centuries ago. This so called "forced feeding" was used in ancient Rome and Greece. Of course the methods used were very primitive at that time. Still, the early medical practitioners saw the need for feeding through an alternative route. Methods and procedures have been refined to benefit the patient that must be fed.

A tube feeding may be necessary for the cancer patient who is unable to eat enough orally to meet the demands of the body and the disease state. Enteral feedings should be initiated immediately when the patient starts to lose weight and has protein losses that cannot be replenished with a regular diet or supplements.

Medical nutritionals through an NG tube

After the patient has been assessed and found to be a candidate for tube feedings, a small tube is placed through the nose and into the stomach for a naso-gastric feeding. Once the tube is placed, liquid medical nutritional products that provide total balanced nutrition are fed to the patient. These feedings can be done comfortably and on an intermittent basis to allow for patient movement during the day. It is very common for tube feeding patients, or their care givers, to learn how to care for the tube and dressing site. Tube feedings are now done on a home basis in large numbers. Naso-gastric tubes are usually inserted only if the feeding will be short term. If the patient is going to require tube feedings for a longer period of time another type of tube may be inserted more suitable for a longer duration.

G tubes defined

The gastrostomy tube may be an alternative to a nasogastric or nose tube, if feedings will be long term. This is often referred to as a "G tube." A gastrostomy is a procedure of placing a tube directly into the stomach, and then feeding the patient by means of the tube. Once again, this procedure will allow the patient to continue to receive all of the nutrients the body needs. You may think of this as giving three well-balanced means a day to the patient, but they are given directly into the stomach. The G tube can be covered by clothing and be inconspicuous. Improved technology now offers tubes that are similar to buttons and that are aesthetically improved.

Placing the G tube

The gastrostomy procedure has been modified within the last several years and can now be placed without surgery. Prior to this time the patient needed to undergo anesthesia and the procedure had to be done in a surgical suite or the operating room of a hospital.

Placement easier and less expensive

The G tube procedure can now be done in an Endoscopy Lab instead of the operating room. This procedure is preferred not only because of the reduced risk to the patient by eliminating anesthesia, but also costs ⅓ of what the surgical procedure would cost. An endoscope is a device with mirrors that, when placed into the stomach, allows for easy placement of the G tube.

The G tube procedure

The endoscope is gently guided down the throat and esophagus. The patient is usually given IV medication to relax them prior to the start of the placement. A small incision is made into the stomach area and the tube inserted. The whole procedure is completed in 30–40 minutes by a well trained surgeon or gastroenterologist. This procedure has been coined the PEG procedure and stands for percutaneous endoscopic gastrostomy.

Feeding through the G tube

Once the G tube has been positioned, feedings can begin through the stomach. With this method, all neccesary needs for protein, calories, vitamins, and minerals can all be given directly into the G tube that bypasses the mouth and throat.

This is an excellent way of keeping large nutritional deficits from occurring early in the therapy period. This procedure could be viewed by the patient as an interim method of eating, and used until the treatment period is finished, and the patient can resume normal eating.

J tubes defined

Another type of tube that can be placed is referred to as a "J tube," and stands for "jejunostomy." When there is a risk of the feeding not staying in the stomach, and the possibility of coming up and going back down into the lungs, a J tube can be used. This situation is called a gastroesophageal reflux, and can result in pulmonary aspiration.

The J tube is done by the same procedure as the G tube, except the tube is placed further down into the intestine. This procedure can be done on an outpatient basis in the GI Lab with an endoscope. With the J tube, the feeding goes directly into the intestine instead of directly into the stomach.

Underutilization of tubes

Both G and J tubes are alternatives that are underutilized with the cancer patient today. Some patients view the procedure of having a tube placed as an effort that reduces quality of life. Recent cases of this type have clouded the benefits that feeding tubes can offer and many patients choose not to have this done. Instead this procedure should be looked at as just one more alternative in the continuum of nutritional feeding that may be only short term until therapy is completed and nutritional deficits remedied.

Is tube feeding beneficial?

Research studies show enteral nutrition has a number of advantages for the immune system with limited risk. New advances in composition of tubes and increased technical advances have established enteral tube feeding as a choice for long term nutritional support of the cancer patient.

Studies show that approximately ⅔ of patients with advanced cancer of the head and neck are malnourished. A recent study at the University of Miami School of Medicine concluded that adequate nutritional support given before cancer therapy will reduce therapy related complications. Benefits of this nutritional support are:

- Patients feel better
- Patients have a higher tolerance to therapy
- Patients have fewer complications
- Patients achieve higher response rates to therapy

Another study at the University of Aberdeen in the United Kingdom evaluated the effect of nutritional support on reducing death in cancer patients undergoing treatment with radiotherapy, surgery, or chemotherapy. The study showed that by giving nutritional supplementation for at least 10 days before surgery, mortality rates were reduced. This study stressed the importance of early intervention because the study showed no evidence that parenteral nutrition (IV), usually initiated after much depletion has occured, prolonged survival.

Parenteral nutrition (Intravenous Feedings)

Parenteral nutrition allows for a more aggressive means of delivering protein, carbohydrates and fat into the system. Parenteral nutrition is often referred to as hyperalementation or "TPN" (total parenteral nutrition.) Typically it is indicated when the gastrointestinal tract is not functioning, or is in need of total rest.

Parenteral means delivery through a vein, and hence total parenteral nutrition is a way for delivering all of your nutritional daily requirements up to 2,500 calories from an IV bottle containing an admixture of protein, carbohydrates, fat, vitamins, minerals, and electrolytes. This concept is considerably different from what is generally delivered in a standard IV bottle of dextrose or saline. Dextrose and saline solutions are indicated primarily for hydration, regulating blood sugar and electrolyte levels, as well as providing a vehicle for administration of medications intravenously. Standard IVs are very important for the above applications, yet provide little with regard to total nutritional requirements.

Early attempts at TPN

The recognized need for alternative feeding methods is not new. The concept of providing nutrients through a vein has actually been around for quite some time. More than a century ago, crude methods were employed in an attempt to accomplish what we do today.

One of the first attempts of TPN was the use of hallowed out chicken bones inserted into veins. Red wine, being recognized as a good source of iron, was funnelled through the chicken bones in an attempt to build the blood. Of course these patients died of infection and did not receive the benefits from the iron.

Since then we have come a long way. We know of a little boy who was born without a gut who has survived over six years on TPN alone. Without TPN he would have died within months. TPN is one of the most exciting nutritional advances in the past few decades.

How is TPN administered? Unlike an IV that is usually started in your arm, the TPN will be infused into a large vein located in the chest area. A local anesthetic is used and only mild discomfort can be felt. This vein is called the superior vena cava. You may already have a catheter in place through which your chemotherapy is given. The device that allows TPN to flow into your body is put into place by a physician and remains there until TPN can be discontinued.

Partial TPN

TPN can also be given on a short-term basis through an IV in the arm. These veins are smaller than the superior vena cava and this route is limited as to the number of calories that can be given.

The TPN mixture can irritate these smaller veins if infused with caloric concentrations that are too high. This is the reason the larger vein is typically used. When this method is employed it is often referred to as "Partial Parenteral Nutrition."

Using TPN in the home

The TPN liquid can be given in the hospital or the patient can be trained to infuse TPN at home. This can be done during the night hours when the patient is sleeping and thereby free the patient during the days hours. Home care nurses can make frequent visits to help with the infusion and check on your bandage changes and answer any questions you may have.

Studies on the use of TPN

Considerable numbers of studies are underway on the bottom line benefits of administering TPN to cancer patients. From a practical standpoint the studies point to the key question of whether the potential benefits of TPN (better tolerance to therapy and improved outcome of therapy) outweigh the potential disadvantages (infection, possibility of feeding the tumor, and possibility of not being able to replete stores to a degree that it would improve outcome.) The studies to date remain inconclusive and controversy continues. Below is a sample of a few of the studies findings.

Dr. Copeland of the University of Texas Medical School in Houston studied 406 patients. In the study 175 patients received both TPN and chemotherapy. Symptoms of vomiting, diarrhea, and nausea were reduced in these patients. Also interesting to note is that 27 percent of the patients had a 50 percent or greater reduction in their tumor mass.

During the American Society for Parenteral and Enteral Nutrition's 13th Clinical Congress Keynote Address, Karyl Richard, Ph.D., of James Whitcome Riley Hospital for Children in Indianapolis spoke to the audience on the pediatric approach to nutritional support. She summarized that "the nutritional state at the time of the diagnosis is related to the outcome. Those who are malnourished at the diagnosis have a poorer outcome compared to the well-nourished." At the same Keynote Address Samuel Klein, M.D., of University of Texas reviewed the topic "TPN and Cancer — Who benefits?" He suggested that TPN may be of benefit "preoperatively in GI tract cancer by decreasing major surgical complications and operative mortality. However no statistically significant benefits from TPN can be demonstrated in survival or tumor response in patients receiving chemotherapy or radiotherapy."

The stance on the efficacy of TPN as an adjunct to cancer therapy varies greatly in the current literature. What we have been able to conclude from dozens of current studies is that early intervention in preventing or correcting nutritional deficits is imperative for a positive outcome. Severe malnutrition is especially dangerous to cancer patients because it narrows the therapeutic margin of safety that exists for responding to repletion with Enteral or Parenteral regimens. When the use of TPN is considered after severe malnutrition has occurred it may not be beneficial enough to warrant its use because of the risks involved with potential infection at the site of the catheter placement.

The reference section will list additional studies done in this area if you are interested in exploring this further.

CHAPTER 5

Basics Of Nutrition

Basic, yes. But simple? Not always. The necessary basics of nutrition range from profoundly simple to quite involved and complex.

Much information available to the general public presents nutrition in simple ways. Yet, many people still ask us, "How does nutrition *really* work?" So settle in and brace yourself for a little studying: this chapter covers the subject in great detail.

You will learn:

- The importance of obtaining calories from a *balanced* source of protein, carbohydrate, and fat.

- Malnutrition is not always visible to the eye, such as in situations of obvious weight loss. Protein is critical. So is sufficient calorie intake in the diet or supplemental feeding. Otherwise, circulating blood proteins are at risk of depletion well before fat stores are broken down. Low blood protein levels (albumin) can seriously impair immune function, compromising the ability to fight off infection.

- The body breaks down lean tissue (such as the delicate muscle that surrounds and protects the heart, lungs and other vital organs) easier than it breaks down excessive stored fat in thighs, hips and stomach when sufficient protein, carbohydrates and fat are not in the diet. Again, this may not be visibly noticeable until the integrity of the system has been seriously compromised, thus hampering recovery. Fortunately, lab tests can readily measure blood proteins (albumin and pre-albumin) so that a physician can assess or predict risk. Monitoring these lab indices regularly makes it easier to intervene with good nutriton to improve or maintain weight and strength, and improve your sense of well-being.

- The importance of fat in the diet: Fat provides more energy per gram than protein or carbohydrates, thereby providing more nutritional momentum at a time when getting enough calories can be difficult. Fat plays many other important roles such as protection of the nervous system, wound healing, maintenance of supple skin, and hormone synthesis. Fat absorbs certain vitamins, such as A, D, E and K. Fat in the diet also reduces stress on the respiratory system.

- By providing an adequate and balanced intake of nutrients, the body will be stronger and may handle more therapeutically effective doses of prescribed chemotherapy and radiation. Again, remember the importance of early intervention with a nutritional maintenance plan.

A short course in basic nutrition

The body can derive energy from three main food components:

1. Protein
2. Carbohydrate
3. Fat

Although chemically distinct from one another, they all have the same function of providing energy for the body. This energy is expressed in terms of calories.

Calories and energy

Some of us associate calories with fat. Actually, a calorie is a measurement of energy. When we consume excessive calories, they store as fat for future energy needs. Calories come from three sources — protein, carbohydrate, and fat. Each one of these components yields a predictable amount of energy (calories) for each gram of intake.

Fat provides more energy than protein or carbohydrate:

- 1 gram of protein supplies four calories
- 1 gram of carbohydrate supplies four calories
- 1 gram of fat supplies nine calories

If calories come from a fat source, the body receives more than twice the fuel for each gram as protein or carbohydrate.

Digestion of Nutrients

The gastrointestinal, or digestive tract breaks down complete substances into smaller, more manageable units. Protein, carbohydrate, and fats break down into their simpler forms, referred to as amino acids, glucose, and fatty acids:

- Protein breaks down to amino acids
- Carbohydrate breaks down to glucose or sugar
- Fat breaks down to fatty acids

These terms are often interchangeable. Before the body can utilize protein, carbohydrate, and fat, it first must convert (digest) them into the simpler forms of amino acids, glucose, and fatty acids. The cell will only be able to utilize the nutrients if they are in this simple, broken-down, "user friendly," form.

Function of nutrients

Although the protein, carbohydrate, and fats of the diet can be used for energy, they are not always used for energy. Sometimes they are used to replace existing body structure, or to add to that structure during periods of growth. For example, some carbohydrates form a part of the supporting or connective tissue of the body, and nerve tissue is composed partly of fats.

Protein is present in the cell walls and makes up much of the interior of the cell. The protein in the cell allows for many chemical processes of the body to proceed efficiently. Cell enzymes are actually proteins.

Although nutrients have multiple functions, all can work to provide energy when the body needs it. A reminder: the body can only use glucose as its sole use of energy, so amino acids and fats held in storage will have to take added steps to convert themselves back into glucose (sugar) when the body needs energy.

How the body creates energy

Carbohydrates are the easiest for the body to utilize, since they break down most efficiently into glucose. Amino acids and fats go through more extensive pathways to convert into glucose so the cell can use it.

Amino acids transform into glucose by a process called "gluconeogenesis." This term literally means "new glucose."

Fat can be converted into glucose, but in a more difficult process. When sufficient glucose is not available for the cell from circulating blood sugar, the body will take the path of least resistance and seek out protein (more easily converted to glucose) to get its energy.

When the body is forced to resort to this, trouble begins, since often the most available protein is the delicate muscle which surrounds and protects the heart, lung, and other vital organs.

What are the nutrients used for once ingested?

Carbohydrates

After a carbohydrate is digested, some of the glucose (sugar) immediately becomes available in the circulating blood for energy. These are the "blood sugar levels" most of us are familiar with.

When the blood attains enough sugar for its immediate needs, some of the glucose stores in the muscle and liver as glycogen. The muscle and liver have limited storage ability, so when these stores fill up, any excess glucose converts into fat.

This excess glucose must take extra steps to get itself back into the "user friendly" form of glucose, should the body call on it for energy later. This is important to remember because the body, if it needs immediate energy, will take the fewest steps to find it by breaking down its protein stores (muscle).

Additionally, blood proteins (i.e., albumin) responsible for immune function are at risk for depletion before fat stores are broken down. This is why early intervention with a nutritional maintenance plan is so important. When the depletion of fat stores is detected, the protein stores probably have been compromised to a great degree, making the patient weaker and less tolerant to therapeutically effective doses of chemotherapy and radiation.

Amino acids

After protein is ingested and broken down to its usable form of amino acids, the body will use it to make up either somatic or visceral protein stores.

61

Somatic protein is "structural" protein. Think of the muscles and connective tissues in your body. Visceral protein is not visible to the naked eye. It is the "circulating blood" protein used for enzyme activity, and, more important, to make antibodies for the immune system.

You will not "see" a depletion of these very important visceral stores. *Thus we underscore the necessity of measuring stores* by lab indices during an initial nutritional assessment, *and monitoring them on a regular basis* to be sure the immune function remains strong during treatments and recovery.

In the early stages of insufficient eating (the first 10 days) the body can more easily tap into protein stores, rather than fat, for its energy. Remember, excessive amounts of glucose (sugar) convert easily to fat, but the reverse — fat to glucose — is not achieved easily.

When available glucose stores are depleted from the blood and liver (two to three days), the body will rely more readily on its protein, rather than fat, for energy. When protein in the body breaks down from its muscle stores, that protein may not necessarily come from the larger arm and leg muscles.

The muscles surrounding your heart, lungs and intestines are at greater risk. So, please note the need for obtaining adequate protein in the diet.

Fats
The body will use fat — broken down into fatty acids — for many vital functions, such as protection of the nervous system, wound healing, maintaining integrity of the skin, and hormone synthesis.

Job completed, excessive amounts of fatty acids store without limit. Fat inclusion in the nutritional plan is vital for two reasons:

    1. To provide calories

    2. To prevent "essential fatty acid deficiency" (EFAD)

Recall that calories from fat provide more energy in each gram than protein or carbohydrate (sugar). Fat is a highly concentrated and efficient source of energy. If the diet lacks sufficient fat, EFAD sets in. The essential fatty acids are:

1. Linoleic acid
2. Linolenic acid
3. Arachidonic acid

All three are essential. However, if linoleic is provided in the diet, the body can manufacture the other two.

Essential fatty acids often are more concentrated in unsaturated fats, such as safflower or sunflower oil. Symptoms of EFAD develop soon if linoleic is missing from the diet. Typically, symptoms manifest on the skin as dry, scaly, eczemous lesions, mostly on the face, palms, soles, and trunk. Left untreated, these lead to sparse hair growth, brittle nails, and more lesions on the skin.

Capillary strength also can be reduced, resulting in easy bruising. More serious complications that affect major organ function will develop if untreated. Other benefits of fat include growth, and biological activities that allow for the absorption of the fat soluble vitamins (A, D, E, and K).

These vitamins can be ingested in the diet, but without the inclusion of fats they will not be absorbed, thereby creating individual vitamin deficiencies. (For example, vitamin K is necessary for blood clotting factors.)

When the patient attempts to meet caloric needs just by carbohydrate (sugar or glucose) and protein (amino acids), and no fat is ingested, the pancreas is stressed. The pancreas's job is to make insulin. Insulin is necessary as a vehicle to carry glucose into a cell. Large amounts of glucose (sugar) in the blood, but not enough insulin, creates the inability for the body to use the glucose. The cell will only accept the glucose if the insulin hand carries it in. The result is hyperglycemia (high blood sugar).

When calories are provided from a balanced source of carbohydrate, protein and fat, the sugar load is not as high, reducing the need for a high amount of insulin. The pancreas then does not have to work as hard.

Research indicates that a balanced diet that includes fat also benefits the respiratory system. Patients who suffer from chronic obstructive pulmonary disease (COPD) must try, by breathing harder, to eliminate the amount of carbon dioxide (CO_2) released as a by-product of ingested food.

The body requires a balance of carbon dioxide and oxygen. Excessive carbon dioxide in the system forces the intake of more oxygen to bring back the balance. This causes more effort to breathe, not only putting strain on the respiratory system, but increasing energy needs even further, thus requiring more calories.

Whereas a healthy individual might burn 80–100 calories a day for breathing, a person with respiratory problems might require 800–1,000 calories a day just for breathing — 10 times more!

You can see why patients with imbalanced nutrition, deficient in fat, usually have tremendous weight loss. They can't keep up with the energy (calorie) needs. The 800–1,000 calories for breathing is over and above the normal daily requirements of 2,000–3,000 calories a day.

Studies on the amount of carbon dioxide produced by each food components — fat, protein and carbohydrate — reveal that carbohydrates give off the highest amount of carbon dioxide. Protein ranks second.

Fats release the least. Patients with respiratory problems offer one of the greatest challenges to nutritonal planning. It's a vicious circle: The body cries out for energy, so . . . increase carbohydrates to meet calorie demands, which . . . increases carbon dioxide in the system, which . . . makes breathing even more difficult.

So, when the lungs labor for more oxygen, a balanced dietary approach that includes more calories from a fat source eases the breathing process, because less carbon dioxide builds up in the system.

This discussion of fat runs a bit more in-depth because it is so misunderstood. Fat has a bad reputation. Often patients raise concerns over the amount of fat in their diet because of the widespread negative attention fat receives. It often is depicted as playing a precursor role in the development of cancer.

But you can see clearly the many good and necessary roles that non-saturated fat can play in the diet of a cancer patient.

While much research indicates that reducing fats in the diet is a good preventative measure for general health, the goal of a person defeating cancer is entirely different. First and foremost, nutritional emphasis shifts to maintaining weight and strength for tolerance of the prescribed treatments.

A balanced approach — inclusive of fats, using them wisely — seems to be the most sensible approach during the period of treatment and recovery.

CHAPTER 6

Devising A Nutritional Care Plan

Plotting a course

Think of a nutritional care plan as a map. Just as a navigator of a boat plots the course to reach a destination, so must a person with cancer map out a plan, commonly known as a nutritional assessment.

This assessment provides information during the treatment therapy and alerts the patient if more aggressive steps are in order to keep the immune system at its optimum.

A map helps only if you have a starting point. Your nutritional starting point is the baseline, and it should be completed immediately after the cancer diagnosis. Evaluating the nutritional status of the patient should be as important as any prescribed chemotherapy, radiation therapy, or surgery.

Typically, the medical world views this suggested path as aggressive behavior, instead of basic medical care. In the medical field nutrition usually is incorporated into the treatment plan too late to have the positive impact that it could have, when started early.

Armed with some fundamental knowledge you can create an interactive role with the health care professionals during treatment, making sure that nutrition is reviewed at every step.

What is a nutritional assessment?

A nutritional assessment consists of different components ranging from questions about your dietary intake to sophisticated laboratory tests. To get an accurate overall picture, an assessment should contain both the formalized lab testing and the less-structured dietary questioning.

Establishing your baseline

To formulate a regimen for nutritional support, first accurately establish the nature and extent of the patient's potential for depletion. This is known as the baseline. It is essential. From the baseline you can determine an individual course needed that will keep the patient at an optimum level of nutritional intake.

Patient interview

Dietary questioning about daily intake and food habits will follow this line of questioning:

- Customary food intake
- Food preferences
- Recent changes in eating habits
- Previous instructions or special modifications
- Religious or ethnic food restrictions
- Typical weight or recent weight fluctuations
- Recent change in appetite
- Recent change in taste or smell
- Difficulty with chewing or swallowing

- Difficulty with digestion of food
- Change in bowel habits
- Food allergies
- Food dislikes or intolerances
- Recent symptoms of nausea or vomiting
- Recent feelings of fatigue, lethargy, or apathy
- Location of tumor and metastases
- Current prescribed drug use
- Vitamin and mineral supplements
- Alcohol use
- Who does food preparation

What is measured in an assessment?

The measurements of the assessment comprises two categories:

1. Anthropometric measurements
2. Laboratory testing

Anthropometrics

Anthropometrics is defined as the measurement of weight, size and proportions of the body, attained through weight, height, and arm measurements for an indication of the amount of fat stored in the body.

Height and weight are the easiest data to collect and are the most useful. The following page details an easy way for estimating desirable weight.

Laboratory tests

Laboratory information coupled with anthropometric measurements provide the most effective method for spotting changes in a patient's nutritional status and response to nutritional support.

ANTHROPOMETRICS

Anthropometrics is defined as the measurement of weight, size and proportions of the body, attained through weight, height and arm measurements for an indication of the amount of fat stored in the body. Height and weight are the easiest data to collect and are the most useful. Below is an easy way for estimating desirable weight.

Height and Weight Table

MEN					WOMEN				
Height		Weight			Height		Weight		
Feet	Inches	Small Frame	Medium Frame	Large Frame	Feet	Inches	Small Frame	Medium Frame	Large Frame
5	2	128–134	131–141	138–150	4	10	102–111	109–121	118–131
5	3	130–136	133–143	140–153	4	11	103–113	111–123	120–134
5	4	132–138	135–145	142–156	5	0	104–115	113–126	122–137
5	5	134–140	137–148	144–160	5	1	106–118	115–129	125–140
5	6	136–142	139–151	146–164	5	2	108–121	118–132	128–143
5	7	138–145	142–154	149–168	5	3	111–124	121–135	131–147
5	8	140–148	145–157	152–172	5	4	114–127	124–138	134–151
5	9	142–151	148–160	155–176	5	5	117–130	127–141	137–155
5	10	144–154	151–163	158–180	5	6	120–133	130–144	140–159
5	11	146–157	154–166	161–184	5	7	123–136	133–147	143–163
6	0	149–160	157–170	164–188	5	8	126–139	136–150	146–167
6	1	152–164	160–174	168–192	5	9	129–142	139–153	149–170
6	2	155–168	164–178	172–197	5	10	132–145	142–156	152–173
6	3	158–172	167–182	176–202	5	11	135–148	145–159	155–176
6	4	162–176	171–187	181–207	6	0	138–151	148–162	158–179

Weights at ages 25–59 based on lowest mortality. Weight in pounds according to frame (in indoor clothing weighing 5 lbs. for men and 3 lbs. for women; shoes with 1-inch heels).

Compliments of MetLife®

Anthropometrics are calculated less frequently than laboratory analysis. Initially, the measurements will be used to set a baseline.

Some lab tests suggesting possible nutritional risk:

- Serum albumin <3.5 g/dL
- Total Lymphocyte count < 1500/mm3
- Hemoglobin <14g/dL in men and <12g/dL in women
- Hematocrit <42% in men and <37% in women
- Reduced Vitamin B12 levels
- Prealbumin (test for reflecting current blood protein) <17 g/dL
- Transferrin (due to short half life reflects current status) <200 mg%

Lab tests defined

Albumin: A protein in human plasma

Total Lymphocyte Count: A lab value derived by multiplying white blood cell count by the percentage of lymphocytes, and dividing by 100

Hemoglobin: The oxygen-bearing protein of red blood cells

Hematocrit: The volume percentage of red blood cells in whole blood

Vitamin B12: A vitamin occurring in foods of animal sources. A lack of vitamin B12 can cause pernicious anemia

Prealbumin: A protein constituent in plasma that determines nutritional status better than albumin because it is not affected as much by fluid status, i.e. dehydration or liver problems

Transferrin: Protein iron binding globulin that facilitates the transportation of iron to the bone marrow and tissue storage area

Complete nutritional assessment

A complete nutritional assessment should include all of the following:

- Dietary History
- Anthropometric measurements: especially height and weight
- Laboratory testing

Other indicators of problems

The body has many ways aside from tests and measurements to naturally reflect early warning signs of malnutrition. Signs and symptoms to recognize that indicate problems:

Face: Dark cheeks and circles under the eyes. Skin on nose and mouth is lumpy or flaky. Face may be swollen.

Hair: Dull, dry, fine, thin, showing lighter or darker spots

Lips: Red and swollen

Eyes: Dull. Eyelid corners are red with bloodshot rings around the cornea.

Teeth: Gums are mushy and bleed easily. Cavities or dark spots appear.

Tongue: Appears swollen with purple sores

Neck: Swollen lymph glands

Skin: Dry, flaky and swollen. Spots resembling bruises appear. Skin appears drawn.

Nails: Brittle, ridged, and spoon shaped

Muscle-skeletal: Wasted muscles, knees bowed, joints swollen, bumps on ribs

Nervous system: Mental confusion and and irritability, and tingling of hands and feet

Internal: Enlarged heart, abnormal rhythm, and high blood pressure. Enlarged liver and spleen.

Why is a nutritional assessment needed?

A nutritional assessment aids the health care professional in evaluating your risk of malnutrition.

Malnutrition exists in two types:

1 protein-calorie malnutrition

2. protein malnutrition

Protein-calorie malnutrition

Protein-calorie malnutrition is the classic very thin person who has probably had a chronic weight loss as well as a loss of muscle. The medical term for this type of malnutrition is "Marasmus."

Protein malnutrition

The appearance of protein malnutrition can be a very subtle. Many times the patient does not look thin and often this form of malnutrition goes undetected. Unlike Marasmus, protein malnutrition may develop very quickly as a result of a disease state that puts metabolic stress on the body. Without protein, the body will begin to cannibalize its own protein stores for nourishment within 2–3 days. Insufficient protein can extend post-operative recovery time, delay wound healing, and increase the risk for complications.

Illustration of malnutrition

If a patient were to ingest 3,000 calories a day from carbohydrate and fat over a long period, his or her body would still break down its own protein stores for the needed protein. The patient might actually gain weight taking in 3,000 calories a day, yet remain malnourished. That's why the caregiver and/or patient must closely review the dietary intake.

In one of our personal case examples, a nurse asked a cancer patient about his appetite. The patient said he had good appetite and the questioning ended there. Later, in the elevator, the patient stated that he was eating mostly fruits.

Therein lies one of the most common myths — call it the "apple-a-day myth": The patient felt like his appetite was strong, and believed he was eating well. Given the increased demands on his immune system, had he continued on a protracted diet of fruits, protein malnutrition would have set in quickly. Indeed, rather than keeping the doctor away, he would have then required even more medical attention, and would have weakened his body's potential for response to it.

Another large misconception among the lay public is that a heavy-set person is nutritionally healthy with "plenty to spare." In reality protein deficits might be present, but not visually detected, thereby putting the heavy and perceived healthy patient as much at risk for malnutrition as the thin, frail individual, as depicted on the opposite page.

Protein balance

Protein is the major nitrogen-containing substance in the body. Measurements of nitrogen can gauge what is happening to the protein in your body. In the normal adult with access to ample food, buildup and breakdown of protein occur simultaneously in a dynamic equilibrium. The buildup balances the breakdown, maintaining proper levels of body protein.

The measure of nitrogen (protein) content of foods ingested

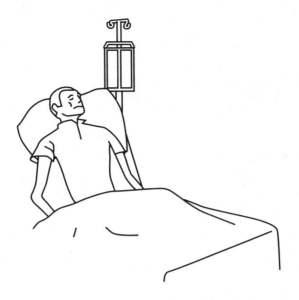

Marasmus: Protein-calorie malnutrition

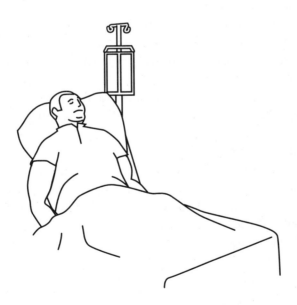

Kwashiorkor: Protein malnutrition

over time, and the measure of nitrogen lost in the urine and the feces in the same period are about equal — known as "nitrogen balance." The body is building up and breaking down protein at equal rates.

Positive nitrogen balance
During periods of growth, the amount of nitrogen excreted tends to be less than taken in. The difference reflects a buildup of protein — called "positive nitrogen balance."

Negative nitrogen balance
When protein malnutrition exists, lost protein exceeds the intake. Sufficiently provided calories help stop the drain on protein stores, but only slightly; protein will still be broken down. This condition is called negative nitrogen balance.

The effects of stress
The cancer patient runs a higher risk of developing negative nitrogen balance because of the stress of the disease. Some of the protein breakdown following a high degree of trauma or surgery is not caused by the inadequate intake of protein; rather, it comes from increased demands of the trauma or disease state. Metabolic stress can cause excessive demands on protein stores.

Higher protein needs
During early stages of starvation, the body burns protein at very high rates of 80–100 grams a day. This is more than a healthy person requires daily. Hence, three balanced meals might not be enough for the cancer patient. The needs are higher because the body is trying to maintain its own stores and repair body tissue as well.

Protein requirements must be calculated with calorie (energy) requirements. A risk is present if protein levels are elevated as well as too low. Both protein and calorie requirements, calculated by a health care professional specifically trained to perform this type of assessment, are extremely important.

Calculating calorie requirements

Two methods of calculating calorie needs:

    1. Indirect calorimetry

    2. Harris-Benedict equation

If indirect calorimetry is unavailable, use this equation — the Harris-Benedict — to determine calorie needs:

Men: (66.4 + 13.7 x weight + 6 x height –6.8 x age)

Women: (655.10 +9.6 x weight +1.8 x height –4.7 x age)

Weight in kilograms

Height in centimeters

Age in years

This formula is the most widely-used for estimating energy requirements.

An easy way to approximate energy needs is to determine your weight in kilograms (divide pound weight by 2.2) and multiply that by 35. Caloric intakes of 30–35 kilocalories are usually adequate to maintain a patient.

Example: A 135-pound woman requires about 2,149 calories, calculated by dividing 135 by 2.2to get 61.4 kilograms, and then multiplying by 35 calories.

Calculating protein requirements

Having calculated calorie needs, you can now figure protein requirements. The recommended dietary allowance of protein for normal healthy adults is 0.8 to 1.0 grams for each kilogram of body weight. Cancer adds metabolic stress to the body and increases the protein needs of the patient. Therefore, requirements might go up to 1.0 to 1.5 or more grams for each kilogram of body weight.

To calculate:

$$\frac{\text{weight in pounds}}{2.2} = \text{weight in kilograms}$$

weight in kilograms x 1.0 or 1.5 grams = daily protein required

A more precise method for determining protein needs is to collect a 24-hour urine specimen and request a lab test called a 24-hour urinary nitrogen test. These formulas provide a general way to estimate calorie and protein needs. The needs vary from patient to patient, depending on the nature and stage of the disease, age of the patient, degree of depletion, etc. The needs assessment should be specific for each patient.

Vitamins and minerals

Requirements for vitamins and minerals are affected by certain disease states, such as cancer. Vitamins and minerals are important in regulating many metabolic processes. Supplemental vitamins should be provided to meet the recommended daily allowance.

The role of minerals is to maintain bone, muscle and nerves. Minerals also play a role in the transformation of energy and fluid balance. Cancer may cause the loss of vitamins and minerals.

Vitamin	Found In	Needed For
A	fish liver oils, green vegetables	Helps fight infection
B1	wheat germ, bran, whole brown rice	Maintains health of nervous system
B2	organ meats — liver, tongue	Maintains muscle tone

B3	poultry, fish, peanuts	Maintains health of digestive system
B5	egg yolks, whole grain cereal	Helps resistance to stress
B6	meats, vegetables, grain products	Needed for red blood cell production
B12	meats, fish, dairy products	Maintains health of nervous system
Biotin	egg yolks, meat, liver, kidney	Deficiency causes fatigue, sleep disorders
C	citrus fruits, vegetables, green peppers	Helps in healing and the production of red blood cells
Choline	egg yolks, liver, wheat germ	Helps nerve transmission
D	egg yolk, fish, fish liver oil	Builds strong bones and teeth
E	green leafy vegetables, eggs, meat	Extends life of red blood cells, protects lungs
Folic Acid	green leafy vegetables, liver	Needed for red blood cell production
Inositol	lima beans, liver, wheat germ	Lowers cholesterol, aids in nervous system
K	egg yolks, leafy vegetables, fruits, meats	Needed for blood clotting
Niacin	liver, lean meats	Involved in oxidative processes
Pantothenic acid	green leafy vegetables, meats	Involved in energy, metabolism

Mineral	Found In	Needed For
Calcium	milk and dairy products	Builds strong bones and teeth
Chromium	meats, whole grain cereal	Aids in carbohydrate utilization
Copper	shellfish, liver, green leafy vegetables	Aids in iron metabolism
Iron	liver, meat, egg yolks	Needed for hemoglobin production
Magnesium	nuts, whole grain	Needed for proper nerve functioning
Manganese	dried fruits, egg yolks	Needed for protein, fat and carbohydrate production
Selenium	broccoli, onions	Protects cells from oxidative damage
Zinc	fish, meats, eggs	Aids in healing

Vitamin RDA (Recommended Daily Allowance)

Vitamin A	Males 5000 IU Females 4000 IU
Vitamin B1 (Thiamine)	1.0 to 1.5 mg
Vitamin B2 (Riboflavin)	1.2 to 1.7 mg
Vitamin B6 (Pyridoxine)	1.6 to 2.0 mg
Vitamin B12 (Cobalamin)	2 mcg
Biotin	100 to 300 mcg
Vitamin C	60 mg
Choline	None established
Vitamin D	200 to 400 IU or 5 to 10 mcg
Vitamin E	8 to 10 IU
Folic Acid	180 to 200 mcg
Inositol	None established
Vitamin K	65 to 80 mcg
Panothenic Acid	10 mg

Calculating fluid requirements

Water intake must also be calculated. Higher amounts of water are required for higher amounts of protein. If water intake is inadequate, dehydration can occur. Generally, the requirements call for one milliliter of water for every calorie consumed. This translates into approximately 2 quarts of fluid a day. If vomiting or diarrhea occur, an electrolyte replacement fluid usually prevents an electrolyte imbalance.

Plotting a nutritional course requires good data collection and a followup plan. Use the following nutritional assessment form; it will be similar to one that a physician is using. The form is not as important as the information that is collected on a consistent, ongoing basis to monitor the patient's nutritional status.

Nutritional Assessment Form

Name: _____

Height: _____

Weight: (Since last visit) _____

(Since diagnosis) _____

Date: _____

Lab Values	Value Reflecting Nutritional Risk	Normal ✓	Abnormal ✓
Prealbumin	<17 g/dL		
Albumin	<3.5 g/dL		
Total Lymphocyte Count	<1500 mm3		
Transferrin	<200 mg%		
Hemoglobin	Men: <14 g/dL Women: <12 g/dL		
Cholesterol	<160 mg/dL		

Questions

	Yes	No
Nausea	_____	_____
Vomiting	_____	_____
Constipation	_____	_____
Diarrhea	_____	_____
Poor appetite	_____	_____
Special diet needs	_____	_____
Number of medications	_____	_____
Problems chewing or swallowing	_____	_____
Skin changes	_____	_____

Physician's Assessment

Check One:

_____ Nutrition Good

_____ Mild Malnutrition

_____ Moderate Malnutrition

_____ Severe Malnutrition

Plan of action:

_____

_____

_____

_____

Date for next assesment to take place: _____

CHAPTER 7

Team Support And Home Care

Home is where the heart is, and it's also where the health is in many cases of cancer care. Most of the time a patient need not lie infirm and eat off a tray, or be tube-fed.

A hospital stay is uncomfortable and expensive. And for many cancer patients it is unnecessary. After initial diagnosis and treatments, doctors admit many patients for the sole reason to assure that they meet their daily nutritional requirements.

Those needs can be handled in the comfort and familiarity — important ingredients for recovery, in and of themselves — of normal surroundings. Home nutritional support is a relatively new concept for providing adequate nutrition. The techniques and methods for feeding have evolved into safe and highly effective ways for treating patients unable to maintain normal nutrition.

With proper training even the patients themselves can administer high-tech feedings, such as enteral and parenteral, which we will explain in a minute.

Growth in home care

In the last decade home health care services have grown tremendously. Advanced medical technologies have paved the way for safe provision of therapies such as home intravenous antibiotic therapy, continuous chemotherapy, pain medication, hydration fluids and nutritional feedings.

Feedings for the home patient

Two types of feedings, parenteral and enteral nutrition, can provide all required caloric and nutrient needs, or a proportionate amount if a patient is able to take some food orally.

Both feedings are versatile — use them either long or short term, alone or in conjunction with one another. A physician will assist in determining which is most appropriate according to individual needs.

Review of parenteral nutrition

Parenteral means "per vein." The method infuses nutrients directly into the blood stream through a plastic tube called a "catheter." Parenteral nutrition can be administered two ways:

1. Total Parenteral Nutritional (TPN)
2. Partial Parenteral Nutrition (PPN)

TPN provides all nutrients necessary for daily requirements. Typically it is used when the patient can't tolerate food, and when the digestive system isn't functioning or needs a rest, precluding enteral tube feedings.

PPN delivers just a portion of the required nutrients through the vein when the patient's digestive system can handle some, but not enough nutrients.

Let's look at the methods separately:

- TPN consists of a mixture of protein, fats, carbohydrates, vitamins, minerals and electrolytes, admixed together in an IV bottle or bag — a simple, ready-for-use form for the cells to take in; no digestion is required. The medical team will instruct you on how to mix these in the home, or they might arrive partially mixed so all you must do is add vitamins and minerals. The mixture can provide 2500 calories or more.

The concentration of the solution requires administering it through a large vein near the heart, permitting rapid dilution of the solution. The volume of the solution would be too irritating and damaging to the smaller, peripheral arm veins.

■ PPN has less volume and concentration, so the smaller, peripheral veins in the arm often tolerate the method.

Supplemental intravenous protein is a typical example of PPN. The therapy assumes that most of the patient's nutrition comes either orally or by tube feedings. The amounts that are not, get replenished by the PPN supplement, which is used primarily to minimize protein losses rather than replace them.

Enteral nutrition

Enteral nutrition is generally considered safer because there is less potential for complications, and it costs less. When the digestive system is functional and oral intake is insufficient, your doctor may choose enteral nutrition — delivering liquid nutrients through a tube that bypasses the mouth.

Oral intake

Many patients lose the pleasure of eating because oral intake was forced on them. They happily forego that experience for a while and rely on the intravenous or tube feedings. This alternate support allows them not only to attain the essential nutritional requirements, but regular eating soon becomes a more pleasurable and enjoyable experience.

If the attending physician allows some oral intake, added amounts of food can be tested gradually. As food tolerance grows, supplemental feedings can be decreased slowly until no longer needed. If the patient holds his or her weight over time and incurs no problems with electrolyte imbalances, they usually can discontinue infusions.

Before starting home therapy, obtain training from a team of physicians, pharmacists and nurses in preparing and administering the feedings selected by the attending doctor.

Insurance coverage

A member of the social service department at the hospital or homecare agency will work with you to secure financial assistance or third-party coverage to help pay for supplies. Fortunately, insurance companies are becoming more receptive to coverage because it eliminates the much higher hospital costs. Medicare's Part B covers enteral and parenteral home therapy when it is the only available source of nutrition. Many times the home care company will handle the billing paperwork.

While the social service person is working on the administrative end, the pharmacist will provide instructions on mixing solutions in the home.

Comfortable learning levels

During the instruction period, a nurse will perform the procedure as you observe and walk through each step. Next, you will carry out the steps with the nurse coaching and supervising. Although the patient usually can self-administer the therapy, whenever possible a family member should become involved in the training session and learn the procedure.

What you will learn

- Principles of sterile technique
- How to care for the catheter site, including daily dressing changes
- How to connect and disconnect the feeding tubes to the catheter
- How to place the heparin lock. (Heparin prevents clotting around the permanent catheter when not in use; it allows for free flow of the feedings.)
- Use of the pump for infusion of fluids
- How to trouble-shoot if problems arise
- How to spot signs and symptoms of complications
- Self-monitoring and record keeping

Team support

A team of health care professionals will follow your progress and be readily available to answer any questions while you are at home. Hospital nutritional support teams coordinate with home care services to provide education, training and followup.

The American Society of Parenteral and Enteral Nutrition has published guidelines and standards of care that are recognized as protocol by most providers of home health care. These standards insure that malnutrition is recognized and treated safely and effectively.

Follow-up

A close patient-physician relationship is important at the beginning of home therapy, and for the duration of therapy.

To assure safe therapy in the home setting, the patient must receive careful monitoring for compliance, adherence to aseptic technique, and screening for possible complications. This entails routine home visits by a registered nurse, as well as periodic follow-up with the doctor.

Placement of the feeding tube

To receive enteral or parenteral feedings at home, the patient undergoes a surgical procedure to place a semi-permanent catheter (tube) in either the vein for parenteral nutrition, or into the digestive system for enteral feedings.

The medical team provides detailed instruction on care of the catheter site and how to attach feedings to the tube. The end of the catheter resembles a plug that can be opened to attach feeding tubes, and closed when not in use.

Intermittent feedings

Unlike many IVs in the hospital that infuse fluids 24 hours a day, nutritional feedings occur intermittently. TPN feedings can be infused during the night, over an 8–10 hour period, leaving the patient free to assume regular daily activities without the tube attached. The catheter site is not cumbersome and can be covered by clothing during the day.

Going home

Once the appropriate type of feeding has been selected, and training on proper procedure for self-feeding is completed, the patient is ready to go home. The care-provider organization will arrange for delivery of supplies to the home. This provider may be either the hospital with its own home health care service, or an agency that specializes in home nutritional support.

Infusion pumps

The supplies include the nutrient mixes, tubing for delivery of the solutions, and an infusion pump (usually electric with battery backup) designed for infusion of the feeding at a constant rate over a specified number of hours.

Failure to maintain an accurate, consistent rate can lead to fluid problems and imbalances in the body's system. The training session includes instruction on use of the pump and an in-depth review of its necessity.

Generally the pump is easy to use. Some have built-in safety and ease-of-use features especially for the home patient. Simple how-to charts provide reference. Pumps usually come equipped with audible and visual alarms that indicate when the feeding is complete, or signal any malfunction. The pump usually attaches to the IV pole. Portable pumps allow mobility for the patient whose feedings take place throughout the day.

Self-mixing at home

You can select from a variety of feeding containers for delivering parenteral or enteral feedings. Parenteral feeding nutrients cannot be fully premixed because of stability problems.

The mixture of nutrients include:

- Amino Acids
- Vitamins
- Dextrose
- Minerals
- Fat
- Electrolytes

A typical way of mixing: combine amino acids and dextrose with the vitamins, minerals and electrolytes all in one bottle or bag. Fat normally is given in a separate bottle that is hooked to the other at the site of the catheter and coinfused. Newer technology allows for mixing all nutrients together in one bag.

With parenteral products it is imperative that you give careful attention to aseptic technique while preparing the solution. Because the products go into a vein, contamination carries the risk of infection. The training pharmacist will thoroughly cover sterile techniques.

Enteral home products

The enteral feedings are considerably easier to self administer. Total nutrition comes in one can. Open it, pour it into the enteral bag, and then hook it up to the catheter for feeding. Newer products on the market come with feedings already in the enteral bag, ready for attachment.

Parenteral feeding risks

Your body is host to microorganisms. Some live there without creating havoc, such as in the path that leads from the mouth to the stomach through the intestines. Other parts of your body are sterile. Blood, for example, is sterile.

If an organism enters a sterile part of the body, infection is likely. Any contaminated item that comes in contact with broken skin surfaces can cause infection. Typical sources of contamination in home nutritional feedings include injection needles, dressings that cover wounds, tubing that delivers solutions, or the solutions.

Use sterile techniques

Your training will stress the sterile techniques necessary for preparing the solutions and caring for the catheter site. With careful attention, there is a smaller risk of an infection. Filters on the IV line trap bacteria before they reach the system. Note that the more effective filters on the market cannot be used on containers that deliver all nutrients through one bag (3-in-1 systems) because the particle size of fat would clog them.

That's an advantage of hanging two bottles, one of fat and the other of protein and carbohydrate. Any bacteria growth by contamination is more likely to take place in the sugar medium of the carbohydrate/protein bottle. The filter of choice by many infection control committees is the smaller .22 micron filter.

With careful attention to preparation of solutions in a clean environment, risk of infection in the home environment is no more than in a hospital.

Our main point is this: avoid becoming lax and careless when preparing feedings just because they are easy and routine.

Enteral feeding risks

The most common risk associated with enteral feedings relates to body tolerance. The most frequent causes of complications are largely prevented by selection of proper formulation, proper determination of rate infusion, and careful monitoring.

Constipation and diarrhea are common side effects occurring from any single factor or combination of factors. Many of the commercial feedings consist of low-residue formulations, and therefore create a decrease in frequency of bowel movements. This should not be confused with constipation.

When constipation occurs, use high fiber feedings. Adequate fluid and exercise will also help. If the problem persists, call the doctor for medication.

Diarrhea might result from bacterial contamination of the feeding solutions. Once the feeding system is prepared and set up in a clean environment, keep it closed. Never add new product to the feeding.

Diarrhea associated with enteral feedings also might occur when fluids enter the body system too rapidly. Your physician might suggest a slower rate of delivery or another product to help alleviate the problem.

Other GI disturbances

Other gastrointestinal upsets include nausea, cramping, and bloating. Generally these problems respond to a 24-hour continuous feeding in which very little solution is introduced into the system at one time.

Self monitoring

To determine whether the home feeding program is providing adequate nutrition and for monitoring problems that arise, collect and record certain information for the attending doctor to review:

Intake/Output

- Record all fluids taken by mouth including soups
- Record all fluids taken from parenteral or enteral feedings
- Record urine output
- Record number of BMs per day
- Notify your doctor if new or increased swelling appears in the feet or ankles

Weight: Weigh each day at the same time. Let the doctor know of any gain or loss of more than 5 pounds a week.

Temperature: Notify a doctor if body temperature rises above 99.6 F for more than 24 hours.

Sugar in the urine: To provide the body with energy, parenteral formulas contain high sugar concentrations. Monitor how well your body is handling the large amounts of sugar. The doctor will provide test tape for measuring sugar in the system. Test for sugar at the end of each infusion, and record the level. Test 6–8 hours later and record again.

Medications: Record all medications and time taken.

Catheter: Look for any redness or drainage, notify doctor if irritated.

Team monitoring

Ongoing and appropriate monitoring by members of the health care team prevents complications and ensures maximum benefits from the nutritional program. If any complication or symptom occurs, notify the doctor immediately. Never alter the rates of infusion without the doctor's instruction.

The team of medical professionals that are working along with you will monitor everything on a regular basis to be sure the prescribed feedings continue to meet the patient's needs most effectively. Medical experts routinely monitor the nutrient intake, review current medications, note signs of intolerances to therapy, weight changes, biochemical and hematological changes, and other signs of nutritional deficiencies and nutrient overloads.

They will notice changes in the patient's life style, and they will help adapt the patient to the new way of "eating." They will assess all major organ functions on a periodic basis.

Who qualifies?

Even if a patient meets all the criteria necessary for receiving enteral or parenteral support, this does not necessarily mean home nutritional support would be best.

Nutritional support is designed to increase the quality of life for a cancer patient in addition to providing the proper food intake. You can see how difficult self-care at home would be for individuals who have little family support, limited dexterity, or little motivation during therapy and treatment. Such a person would have difficulty in complying with the many steps required for successful home support.

If, on the other hand, the patient is fortunate to have a supportive home environment and his or her condition is medically stable, home nutritional support probably provides a desirable alternative. The patient and family or friends, sufficiently motivated and capable of learning procedures for safe feeding at home, can then offer the enhanced quality of life that comes with normal daily routine. Home support allows for independence and control, for returning sooner to a prehospitalized role, and for restoration of self esteem and a sense of well-being.

Who decides?

The decision for home nutritional support cannot be made by either the attending doctor or the patient unilaterally. Both must evaluate the suitability and desirability of home therapy. The doctor and the health-care team must explain thoroughly the risks and benefits of selected nutritional therapy in the home setting.

Home nutritional support represents an exciting option for those who require more aggressive nutritional management. It is cost-effective and practical. Home nutritional support gives these patients the opportunity to take advantage of optimum nutrition without having to starve first to qualify for treatment.

We can't stress it enough: Ask questions. Persist with the medical team to address your nutritional program. With your list of questions in hand, request this information.

CHAPTER 8

Putting It All Together

We have given you a plethora of information about nutrition and the benefits of nutritional intervention. All of this knowledge will be useless unless assimilated into a workable and understandable plan for the individual patient.

First, you must understand the importance of *your* role in taking charge of nutrition in the battle against cancer. Even though nutrition is very basic, many times a medical team will not address nutritional care as early as necessary for it to have a positive impact on the outcome.

You may have to initiate the subject of nutrition and press for how it will be integrated into treatment at the earliest stage. We hope that with this knowledge you can facilitate an interactive role with your physician. You must be assured that nutrition will be addressed from the first visit.

Prevalence of malnutition

Often people think that malnutrition is something found in Third World countries among starving children with protruding bellies. Medical studies undertaken in the United States documented in 1974 that the rate of malnutrition in our hospitals ranges from 35–50 percent. With this problem identified more than 20 years ago, why, with all of our scientific technology, hasn't this issue been addressed and explored further? Sadly, these statistics still hold true.

Why hasn't the condition improved? We believe it's simply because nutrition is not addressed until too late. Nutrition is so basic that many times it is just taken for granted or completely overlooked.

Winston Churchill once said, "Men occasionally stumble on the truth, but most of them pick themselves up and hurry off as if nothing happened."

Because of heavy, demanding course loads, medical schools do not focus on nutrition as much as specific disease states. Recently, we heard an oncology researcher in dismay over how little headway we have made in the war against cancer. While nutrition can't cure cancer, studies show that it can have a *positive impact on outcome if implemented early.* Our mission is to increase nutrition awareness both among the medical profession as well as through cancer patients and their caregivers.

We continually talk with cancer patients about what they have been told to do nutritionally, and far too many times we learn that they have not been given any instruction.

The challenge lies before you: initiate a conversation about nutrition at the first meeting with the physician. Take heart that there are many positive steps available for nutrition.

STEPS TO TAKE
Cancer Diagnosis
Getting a Nutritional Assessment

Nutrition Good

↓

Continue getting
enough calories and
protein and recheck
every 2–3 weeks

Unable to Eat

↓

Have a J or G tube
placed if the GI is
functioning (Enteral
Nutrition)

↓

IV Nutrition
(Parenteral Nutrition)

**Nutrition Deficits
Exists**

↓

Able to eat

↓

Supplement regular
meals with nourish-
ments or medical
nutritionals

↓

Continue to recheck
nutrition weekly

Questions to Ask Your Physician Regarding Your Nutrition

✓ Who will be in charge of evaluating my nutritional status initially? (i.e., Physician, Dietitian or Nutritionist, IV Nurse, Hospital Nutritional Support Team)

✓ Who will be in charge of evaluating my nutritional assessment on an ongoing basis? (i.e., Oncologist, Internist, Family Practice Physician)

✓ What will the assessment measure and who will keep the records?

✓ Where will the assessment be done? (i.e., Dietary Office, Lab, Physician Office, Hospital)

✓ When will the initial assessment of my nutritional status take place?

✓ How often will it be re-assessed?

✓ Who will be responsible for consulting with me on the final plan?

✓ What educational resources are available regarding my nutrition?

Cooking for Your Health

While putting together the following recipes we tried to be mindful of what would be helpful if: (a) you were not feeling well physically or had special concerns that made eating difficult such as mouth sores, dry mouth, or difficulty swallowing, (b) you were tired and had to prepare the food yourself, and (c) you were feeling emotionally down and had a hard time motivating yourself to really care about food.

Our sampling of recipes include easy to prepare, as well as more involved for instances where a caregiver may be helping prepare the food. Regarding the theme of selections, we purposely did not settle in on one tone. One minute we speak of tofu, and the next . . . Twinkies. It is our experience that different things work for different people and while one minute you may want nothing but whole, fresh foods that satisfy, sustain, enliven; other times a Hostess cupcake is what will really do the trick. When dealing with such an imperative to maintain body weight against the odds of doing so, immediately the goal is do what it takes (in moderation of course)

101

to get the calories in. If a sufficient balanced diet cannot be tolerated at this time, there are options as discussed in this book, no need to feel guilty that you are not eating just the right food. Supplemental protein can be given throughout the day in sips from fortified drinks, or if necessary from enteral or parenteral nutrition as discussed.

Although we have been stressing higher caloric and protein selections throughout the book, the recipes do include a number of low calorie selections, especially in the fruit area. This inclusion is to balance out the diet. Fruits are an important source of vitamins, minerals, fiber and micronutrients, and fruit can be quite refreshing when richer, nutritionally dense food may be unappealing. Also, fresh seasonal fruits can be uplifting emotionally. Think of how the fuzzy down on a fresh peach feels, or how the sight of jewel tone pomegranate seeds sprinkled over banana slices look, or the smell of fresh green apples when being sliced. Letting your other senses come into play during mealtime can enhance the experience in unexpected ways.

Meanwhile, listen to your body and see what will work for you with the most degree of comfort during the times when getting enough is difficult. Again we stress, if you cannot ingest enough orally to meet your increased needs, *don't wait for weight loss to occur before asking for assistance with your diet.*

To your good health,

Jane and Susan

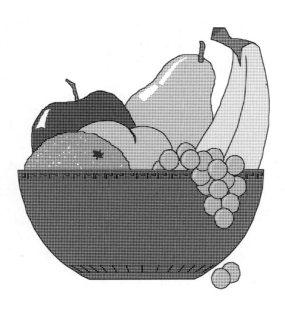

Menu and Recipes

MENU

Fortified Drinks

French Fiber Fantasia
Alpine Delight
Almond Nectar
Mock Egg Nog

Breakfast/Dinner

Maple and Cinnamon French Toast
Tangerines and Brown Rice Cereal
Warm Buckwheat Kasha Cereal
Asparagus and Mozzarella Omelet
Pita Pockets with Garbanzo Bean Salad
Roast Chicken and Watercress
Pumpernickel, Provolone, Tuna Melt
Crock Pot Lasagna
English Broccoli and Cheese "Pasties"

Soups

Chicken Noodle Soup
Cream of Celery Soup
Corn and Potato Chowder
Chilled Creamed Cucumber Soup

Casseroles and Side Dishes

Fortified Green Bean Casserole
Easy Cheesey Potatoes
Hashbrown Casserole Bake

Mini-meals and Snacks
Cucumber Raita Dip with Pita Bread
Apples Dipped in Nut Butter

Fresh Fruit Entrées
Nectarines and Blackberries
with thinly sliced Swiss on the side
Fresh Sliced peaches, Plumbs and Boysenberries
with Almond Butter Cookies
Sliced Oranges, Strawberries and Red Grapes
with Wheat Toast
Lemon Sherbet and Blackberries with Gingersnaps
Blackberry Sorbet and Red Raspberries
Raspberry Sorbet with Sliced Plumbs and Mint Sprigs
Sliced Mangoes with Ginger and Lime Zest

Desserts
Lime Ice Pops
Popsicle Slush
Gingerbread
Key Lime Pie with Kiwi Fruit
Lemon Shortbread and Cherries
Blueberry Cobbler
Peach Yogurt Gelatin

French Fiber Fantasia

> 1 8-ounce can Vanilla Supplement with Fiber (can liquid protein supplement)
> 1 packet French Vanilla Instant Breakfast
> 1 cup of milk
> 1 Hostess cupcake

Mix all ingredients in blender for 30 seconds. Chill.

High protein content: 22 grams

Alpine Delight

> 1 8-ounce can of Chocolate Supplement
> 1 packet French Vanilla Instant Breakfast
> 1 packet Swiss Miss Cocoa Mix
> 5 medium strawberries
> ½ teaspoon almond extract

Mix all ingredients in blender for 30 seconds. Chill.

High protein content: 16 Grams

Almond Nectar

1 **8-ounce can Vanilla Supplement**
1 **Almond Joy candy bar**
⅓ **cup marshmallow creme**

Mix all ingredients in blender on high 30 seconds. Heat
mixture in the microwave 1 minute. Add ½ teaspoon vanilla
extract.
High protein content: 10 grams

Mock Egg Nog

1 **8-ounce can of Egg Nog Flavored Supplement**
4 **ice cubes shaved or crushed**
½ **teaspoon grated nutmeg**
¼ **teaspoon almond extract**

Crush ice in blender, add liquid eggnog supplement and
almond extract. Pour in glass and sprinkle with nutmeg.

*Armchair note: The smell of nutmeg can be a real treat for the senses,
helping to coax a sense of well-being.*

Maple Cinnamon French Toast

4 slices whole wheat bread
2 eggs
¼ cup whole milk
2 tablespoons pure maple syrup
¼ teaspoon ground cinnamon

Syrup
¼ cup pure maple syrup
1 tablespoon melted butter
½ teaspoon fresh grated orange zest

Melt small amount of butter in fry pan. Whisk eggs in bowl, add milk, syrup and cinnamon. Dip bread in egg mixture and grill both sides in pan. Heat syrup ingredients on low, pour over toast and serve.

Armchair note: French Toast can be a great dinner meal. Easy, satisfying and complete.

Tangerines and Brown Rice Cereal

  1 **cup short-grain brown rice**
  2 **cups soy milk (*not* the fat free variety)**
  ½ **cup of water**
  1 **teaspoon grated fresh orange rind**
  ½ **teaspoon grated nutmeg**
  2 **tangerines, peeled and sectioned**

Combine rice, soy milk and water in a bowl the night before
(to reduce cooking time next morning) and keep refrigerated.
Next morning bring mixture to a boil, reduce and simmer for
15–20 minutes, stirring occasionally until liquid is absorbed
and rice is soft. Serve in bowls with nutmeg, tangerine sec-
tions and orange rind as garnish.

*Armchair note: Soy milk makes for easier digestion if having a
problem with lactose intolerance. It also makes a creamier hot cereal
than whole milk. If you have a crock pot, put all in the night before
with the exception of the tangerines and set on low. Eight hours later
in the morning it will be ready.*

Warm Buckwheat Kasha Cereal

**1 cup of roasted buckwheat kernels (Kasha),
    available at most health food stores**
1 egg
2 tablespoons butter
1½ cup water
**1 teaspoon maple syrup or honey
    Milk, raisins or chopped dates to taste**

Mix egg and kasha together well in bowl. Melt butter in pan and sauté buckwheat kasha 3–4 minutes Add water, heat to a simmer and reduce heat, cook for 10–15 minutes. Add syrup or honey if sweetness desired. Add soy or whole milk with chopped raisins or dates.

Armchair note: Kasha is one of Russia's core comfort foods. It is a hearty, rather bland grain. This porridge of roasted buckwheat is a typical Russian breakfast.

Asparagus and Mozzarella Omelet

2-3 eggs
3 ounces of mozzarella cheese
3-4 fresh asparagus (steamed until tender)
½ teaspoon olive oil
½ teaspoon butter
¼ teaspoon oregano (crushed)
Salt and pepper to taste

Melt olive oil and butter in omelet pan. Whisk eggs and add to pan. As eggs start to firm, place asparagus on top and sprinkle with mozzarella and oregano. Cook until cheese melts and fold over. Good served with pumpernickel toast.

Armchair note: Many culinary herbs are used not only for flavor, but have carminative properties as well in that they gently aid in digestion. One such herb is oregano.

Pita Pockets with Garbonzo Bean Salad

    1 **can of garbonzo beans (chick-peas), rinsed and drained**
    ⅓ **cup fresh chopped parsley**
    3 **tablespoons lemon juice**
  1½ **tablespoons olive oil**
    1 **garlic clove, minced (if desired)**
    ¼ **cup red onion thinly sliced**
    ½ **cup diced cucumber**
    3 **cups soft lettuce greens (such as bib lettuce)**
    ½ **cup plain yogurt (full fat variety)**
    ¼ **teaspoon ground cumin**
 3–4 **Pita shell pockets**

Mix first 5 ingredients together in bowl. Then lettuce, cucumber, and onion to bowl and toss. Mix yogurt and cumin to be used as a dressing. Fill pita pockets with mixture and top with yogurt dressing.

Armchair note: In India cooks use warming blends of spices and herbs to stimulate digestion. Cumin is often used as a balancing herb and tonic for the system.

Crock Pot Lasagna

1 large jar of prepared tomato sauce
1 8-ounce package of uncooked lasagna noodles
8 ounces ricotta cheese
8 ounces firm tofu, drained and mashed
1 cup broccoli, chopped
½ cup sliced green zucchini
½ cup sliced yellow squash
½ cup sliced mushrooms
1 pound pre-grated mozzarella (soy mozzarella if you
   have lactose intolerance problems)
¾ cup fresh fine-grated Parmesan cheese
½ teaspoon crumbled basil

Spray crock pot with nonstick spray for easy clean up. Pour ⅓ of tomato sauce on bottom of crock pot. Break noodles to fit in a layer. Layer half of the vegetables, ricotta, tofu, and mozzarella. Top with another ⅓ of sauce. Repeat with layer of noodles, rest of vegetables, ricotta, tofu, mozzarella. Final layer of noodles and sauce. Top with parmesan. Cook on low for 7–8 hours, or high for 3–4 hours. Serve with French bread and green salad.

Armchair note: Crock pots can be a real help when you want to eat but don't want to cook and may not have the option of someone preparing your meal. Put your crock pot in the garage or on the back porch and voila! No cooking odors, easy casseroles and stews and little clean up. Crock pots can run $12–$15 and often come with their own how-to booklet inside.

English Broccoli and Cheese "Pasties" (English Pub Hand Sandwiches)

1 head of broccoli, cut into florets
8 ounces mild cheddar cheese, grated
2–3 tablespoons finely diced chives (milder than green onions)
1 tablespoon finely chopped fresh dill
⅛ teaspoon ground nutmeg
2 ready-to-serve pie crusts (2 to a box; found in refrigerated section of grocery store)
1 egg beaten with 1 tablespoon of water (for glaze)

Preheat oven to 400°. Steam broccoli florets and mix into bowl with cheese, chives, dill and nutmeg. Unfold the 2 pie crusts on counter and cut circles in half so you have 4 half circles. Fill each with a ¼ of mixture.

Press filling in tight and fold over circle creating a triangle pocket. Use fork to tightly crimp edges. Put on cookie sheet and brush with egg glaze. Bake 20 minutes and let set for 5 minutes. Serve with red grapes.

Armchair note: The herb dill comes from the Norse word "dilla," meaning to lull. The lacy blue green herb is rich in minerals and has relaxing properties, often it is used as a digestive aid. Freshly chopped, it has a distinctive tang that can stimulate the appetite and it is often used in soups and complements most fish nicely.

Breakfast/Dinner

Pumpernickel, Provolone, Tuna Melt

1 can tuna in spring water (less fish odor than the oil variety)
1 tablespoon Mayonnaise
1 teaspoon fine-chopped onion
1 tablespoon fine-chopped celery
⅛ teaspoon garlic powder (optional)
⅛ teaspoon celery seed
2 slices provolone cheese (smoked or regular)
2 slices pumpernickel toast

Mix first 6 ingredients in bowl and mix well. Divide onto two pieces of pumpernickel and top with provolone cheese. Broil until melted. Serve open-faced with red grapes on the side.

Roast Chicken and Watercress

1 small warm rotisserie-roasted chicken (typically found precooked in the deli section of large grocery stores)
1 bunch fresh watercress
1 commercial bottle of quality, mild vinaigrette

Rinse watercress, pat dry and arrange on platter. Place precooked chicken on top (reheat if necessary) and drizzle chicken and watercress with vinaigrette.

Armchair note: Watercress is not always available, however when it is, you're worth the splurge. Also buy precooked rotisserie chickens when available and use leftovers for sandwiches and in salads to boost protein intake.

Chicken Noodle Soup

- 1 **4-pound roasting chicken**
- ½ **onion, thinly sliced**
- 1 **carrot cut into half moons**
- 3 **parsley sprigs**
- 1 **teaspoon salt**
- 1 **teaspoon white pepper**
- 2 **medium russet potatoes, pealed and thinly sliced**
- 1 **celery stalk with leaves, thinly sliced**
- 2 **thyme sor ½ teaspoon dried thyme**
- 1 **package egg noodles**

Put chicken in pot with enough cold water to cover. Add next 5 ingredients. Bring to a boil, reduce heat to a simmer and cook 1 hour. Remove chicken, let cool and remove meat. Skim off excess fat from top of broth. Add potatoes, celery and thyme to broth, bring to a boil until potatoes are tender, about 15 minutes. Add noodles until tender. Serve.

Armchair note: If you are not feeling well and someone is unavailable to make this for you, use the following shortcut.

Bring 3 cans of chicken broth to a boil with onion, carrot, parsley and potatoes. Cook for 15 minutes until potatoes are tender. Add celery, thyme, pieces of precooked rotisserie chicken. Add wonton wrappers cut into 2-inch squares (they taste like homemade noodles!), and cook an additional 8 minutes.

Cream of Celery Soup

1 can of cream of potato soup
1 cup milk
1 stalk celery with leaves, finely chopped
¼ teaspoon celery seed

Heat together in sauce pan. Ladle into bowl and serve with rye bread.

Corn and Potato Chowder

1 tablespoon butter
½ onion, finely chopped
½ pound red-skinned potatoes, peeled and diced
2 cups frozen corn
2 cups half-and-half
1 cup chicken broth
½ teaspoon crumbled marjoram
2 cups grated mild white cheddar cheese

Melt butter in sauce pan and sauté onion 5 minutes. Add potatoes, corn, half-and-half, broth and marjoram. Slowly add cheese until melted. Serve with whole grain bread.

Chilled Creamed Cucumber Soup

> 2 tablespoons olive oil
> 2 shallots, finely chopped (lighter in taste than onions)
> 1 garlic clove, finely chopped (optional)
> 4 large cucumbers peeled, seeded and chopped
> ½ cup whipping cream
> 2 tablespoons white balsamic or white wine vinegar
> ⅛ teaspoon white pepper

Heat oil in sauce pan and sauté shallots and garlic until tender, approximately 5 minutes. Transfer to food processor. Add cucumbers and purée. Add cream and vinegar pulsing on and off. Strain soup through a sieve, add pepper, chill overnight.

Armchair note: Chilled soups are especially soothing for dry and irritated mouths often a side effect of the treatments. Many recipes for chilled soup are available, look through cookbooks and see what agrees.

Fortified Green Bean Casserole

1 can cream of mushroom soup
½ can Vanilla Supplement (canned liquid protein drink)
1 teaspoon soy sauce
2 8-ounce cans green beans, drained
1 can french-fried onions

Combine first 3 ingredients in a buttered 1½-quart casserole
dish. Add the green beans and stir in half of the onions. Bake
350° for 30 minutes. Add the rest of the onions and return to
the oven for 5 minutes.

Easy Cheesy Potatoes

8 ounces sharp cheddar cheese
8 ounces sour cream
4 cups hashbrown potatoes

Mix together and bake at 350° for 25–30 minutes.

Hashbrown Casserole Bake

3 cups frozen hashbrowns
⅓ cup melted butter
1 pound bacon, cooked and crumbled
2 cup canned mushrooms, drained
½ cup milk
3 eggs, beaten

Spread hashbrowns into bottom of lightly greased 13x9x2
baking dish. Drizzle the melted butter over. Mix bacon,
mushrooms and half of the cheese and spoon mixture over
hashbrowns. Combine eggs and milk and pour over mixture.
Top with remaining cheese. Bake 350° 25–30 minutes.

Cucumber and Raita Dip with Pita Bread

  1 **large cucumber (peeled and seeded)**
  1 **tablespoon, finely minced onion (optional)**
1½ **cups yogurt (plain, full-fat variety)**
  ¼ **teaspoon cumin (Indian spice)**

Grate or finely chop in food processor the peeled and seeded cucumber. Add cumin to 2 tablespoons of yogurt and heat slightly until spice is blended. Stir together the cucumber, onion, yogurt and cumin mixture in bowl and serve as snack with pita bread wedge for scooping up dip.

Armchair note: This Indian side dish is very cooling and soothing to the mouth. It's a refreshing snack that is somewhat different yet bland.

Apples Dipped in Nut Butters

Slice apples and dip in a variety of nut butters. Larger varieties of butters available in health food stores. A good one to try is almond butter (looks like peanut butter).

Armchair note: Nut butters can be made fresh by putting nuts and seeds through a hand baby food grinder (inexpensive and available in most health food stores and catalogs.)

Hint!

A good source for whole, fresh foods and baked goods that will deliver to your home is: Walnut Acres Organic Farms, Penns Creek, PA 17862, 1-800-433-3998 (call for catalog).

Using Walnut Acres' home delivery service (UPS), you don't have to load and unload the car (a big plus if you have had any surgery, don't feel well, or have little help), and the delivery charges are very reasonable, in fact less expensive than the cost of many local grocery delivery services.

Their raspberry crunch granola and cinnamon sticky buns are terrific. This catalog and its services make life easier when you have little help grocery shopping and preparing meals for yourself or family.

Fresh Fruit Entrées

This section is a listing of fruits that look pretty and complement each other nicely. When shopping for fruit try to buy what is in season as it is usually the best in quality with regards to freshness, natural sweetness and color. For ease of preparation buy good quality commercially prepared side treats such as gingersnaps and almond butter cookies.

We feast with our eyes before we taste with our taste buds. Visual ambiance makes all the difference. The pattern of the tablecloth and the color of the service pieces can affect the whole gustatory experience. Flowers on the table can set the tone for mood. You don't need big bouquets or arrangements. Try 2 or 3 little antique medicine bottles on the table filled with a few wildflower stems. Color is relaxing and it stimulates and appetite. Consider the soothing effects of cool blue and purple Veronica flowers with a sprig of Queen Anne's Lace, or the cheery bright colors of red Poppies, or the loveliness of white Gardenias, or the simplicity of earthy greens such as ivy.

Below are some suggestions for fruits that work synergistically well together. Anything that appeals to you will work, use your imagination. Contrast texture and color. Use simple china if the colors of the food are to be the focal point, don't use overly ornate dishes that end up competing with the food.

Nectarines (sliced) and blackberries
serve with thinly sliced and rolled Swiss cheese

Fresh sliced peaches, plumbs and boysenberries
serve with almond butter cookies on the side

Sliced oranges (peel and rind removed), strawberries and red grapes
serve with wheat toast

Lemon sherbet and blackberries
serve with gingersnaps

Blackberry sorbet and red raspberries
serve with waffle cone cookies

Raspberry sorbet with sliced plumbs (skin on) and fresh mint sprigs
serve with slices of thin plain pound cake on the side

Sliced mangos (skin off) sprinkled with candied ginger and lime zest*

* *Crystallized or "candied" ginger offers a slightly unusual taste and texture. Fresh ginger is cured in sugar, packaged sliced, and coated with a coarse sugar. It is typically imported from Australia.*

Lime zest will give the fruit a tartness and an intensely aromatic flavor. Grate the green rind , but not the white pithy part underneath. It's pretty and flavorful, the same can be done with lemons and oranges.

Lime Ice Pops

1 small can of frozen lime concentrate
Water for mixing

Mix the frozen concentrate with *half* the suggested water on the
can. Freeze the juice in plastic popsicle forms (found in the
grocery store), or in an ice cube tray. Suck on for snacks.

Armchair note: The tartness of the lime helps stimulate saliva produc-
tion and the sweetness may help offset nausea. If mouth sores are a
problem you may want to avoid citrus.

Popsicle Slush

1 popsicle, any flavor
¼ cup of 7-Up

Pour soda in a cup, add popsicle and microwave for 10–15
seconds (or until a slush consistency). Remove stick and eat
with a spoon in cup.

Armchair note: This one is great for nausea. A nurse in a Dallas
hospital recovery room shared this one with me, they use it for first
oral fluids after surgery. Simple and it works.

Gingerbread

      3 cups all-purpose flour
      1 tablespoon ground cinnamon
      1 teaspoon ground cloves
      1 teaspoon ground ginger
     ¼ teaspoon allspice
     ¾ teaspoon salt
      2 teaspoon baking soda
   1½ cups sugar
      1 cup vegetable oil
      1 cup unsulfured molasses
     ½ cup of water
   1½ tablespoons fresh grated ginger

Preheat oven to 350°. Sift first 7 ingredients into large bowl.
Blend well the next 5 ingredients in another bowl. Transfer dry
ingredients into liquid mixture. Pour batter into buttered and
floured 10″ pan. Bake approximately one hour, cool one hour.

*Armchair notes: Brighten plain, dark baked goods with a light
snowy sifting of confectionery sugar. Ginger is often taken to offset
motion sickness. Gingerbread is wonderfully settling to the stomach.*

Key Lime Pie with Kiwi Fruit

      2 cans of sweetened condensed milk (15–16 ounces)
      4 egg yolks
      6 ounces key lime juice (unsweetened)
    1–2 sliced kiwi fruit, skin cut off
      1 graham pie crust, pre-made in pie shell

Mix yolks into condensed milk, whisk in Key lime juice. Pour into prepared pie crust. Bake 350° 15 minutes. Chill. Decorate top with sliced kiwi.

Lemon Shortbread with Cherries

    1¼ all-purpose flour
     ¼ cup of sugar
      1 stick of unsalted butter, cut into pieces
      1 tablespoon fresh lemon juice
      1 tablespoon lemon peel, finely grated
     ⅛ teaspoon nutmeg

Sift flour and sugar into bowl, work in butter by hand, add lemon juice, peel and nutmeg. Work dough until it sticks together. Put dough on floured surface and break into two balls. Put each ball on greased baking sheet and flatten out each to 5″ rounds. Pierce holes all over dough with a fork, and crimp edges with a fork for decoration. Score each round into six wedges. Bake 300° for 50 minutes. Cut wedges and cool.

Dust shortbread lightly with powdered sugar, and serve with cherries and a cup of tea.

Blueberry Cobbler

    4 **cups blueberries (or 16 ounces unsweetened package)**
    ¾ **cup brown sugar**
    1 **stick of unsalted butter, cut into small pieces**
    1 **cup all-purpose flour**
    1 **cup milk**
    1 **egg**
    ¼ **cup uncooked-cooked oats**
    ½ **teaspoon vanilla**
    1 **teaspoon dried orange peel (in the store by the spices)**

Put blueberries in greased pie dish, coat berries with 1 table-spoon of flour and ¼ of the brown sugar. In a bowl mix remaining flour and butter to form a coarse meal. Mix in remaining brown sugar, oats, milk, egg, vanilla and orange peel. Pour batter over berries. Cook at 350° for 55 minutes. Let cool. Serve with ice cream .

Peach Yogurt Gelatin

    2 **cups of peach juice (found in health food stores,**
          or use tropical blends found in grocery stores)
    1 **package unflavored gelatin (such as Knox)**
    8 **ounces plain yogurt (full fat variety)**
    1 **teaspoon honey**

Bring half of the juice to a boil and add gelatin. Remove from heat and add remaining one cup of juice. When the gelatin begins to set, stir in yogurt and honey. Chill until firm.

Cancer Survivors Guide

Who is a cancer survivor? Anyone who has ever been diagnosed with cancer and is alive today is a Survivor!

The art of "survivorship": Every Survivor has the right to pursue the best quality of life possible after a cancer diagnosis by addressing those issues which affect that quality. A good place to start is to acquire as much cancer-related knowledge as possible, and to interact with support groups.

What is cancer? Cancer is a group of over 100 diseases characterized by the uncontrolled growth of abnormal cells in the body. Normal cells become abnormal when they are exposed to carcinogens such as radiation (for example, ultraviolet rays of the sun) or particular drugs or chemicals. They can also turn malignant (cancerous) when they are attacked by certain viruses or when some not yet fully understood internal signal occurs. Once cells become malignant, they multiply more rapidly than usual. Then they often form masses called tumors that invade nearby tissue and interfere with normal bodily functions. Cancer cells also have a tendency to spread to other parts of the body, where they form a secondary tumor.

Cancers are classified according to the type of cell and the organ in which they start:

- **Carcinoma,** the most common kind of cancer, arises in the epithelium, the layers of cells covering the body's surface or lining internal organs and various glands.

- **Melanoma,** an increasingly prevalent form of cancer, starts in pigment cells located among the epithelial cells of the skin.

- **Sarcomas** originate in the supporting (or connective) tissues of the body, such as bones, muscles, and blood vessels.

- **Lymphomas** are born in the cells of the lymph system — the body's circulatory network for filtering out impurities.
  Within these broad classifications, cancers are often divided into more specific categories based on cell subtype and affected organ.

Cancers are also classified in terms of how far they have spread, and to what organs:

- **An in situ** cancer has spread to surrounding tissues.

- A **metastasized** cancer has invaded distant sites in the body.

In diagnosing cancer, doctors take all these aspects of classification into account to arrive at a decision on what type of cancer a patient has and what stage it's in. Proper diagnosis and treatment rely on accurate classification.

Investigational treatments and clinical trials

Investigational treatments are promising means of treating cancer that are still in the testing stages. The testing is done in highly regulated and carefully controlled patient studies called clinical trials, many of which are sponsored by the National Cancer Institute.

All clinical trials must follow a specific protocol, or plan, that is designed to answer specific questions and guard a patient's health and well-being. Patients are admitted to a clinical trial only if their medical condition meets the specifics of the protocol.

Clinical trials are conducted in four separate phases, aimed at discovering certain types of information about treatment in question:

- **Phase I** trials are meant to determine safe dosage and side effects. They are conducted with a small number of patients, and only people with advanced cancer who cannot be helped with standard treatments take part.

- **Phase II** trials seek to gauge the effectiveness of a treatment for different types of cancer.

- **Phase III** trials compare new treatment with the best known standard treatment(s) to decide which is better.

- **Phase IV** trials establish the new treatment as a standard therapy for patient use.

No treatment moves from one phase to the next unless it proves its potential in the previous phase. Patients in clinical trials have the first opportunity to benefit from new treatments. Participation is voluntary from the start of a trial to its finish — a patient can drop out at any point and receive the best known standard therapy.

American Brain Tumor Association
2720 River Road, Suite 146
Des Plaines, IL 60018
800-886-2282
Offers free services including publications about brain tumors, support group lists, referral information and a pen pal program

American Cancer Society (ACS)
1599 Clifton Road NE
Atlanta, GA 30329
800-ACS-2345
  Reach to Recovery
  I Can Cope
  Road to Recovery
  International Association of Laryngectomees
  Look Good, Feel Better
  Resources, Information & Guidance (RIG)
Dedicated to eliminating cancer as a major health problem through research, education, and service

American Foundation for Urologic Disease
300 West Pratt Street, Suite 401
Baltimore, MD 21201
800-242-2383
  Bladder Health Council
  Prostate Health Council
  Prostate Cancer Survivors Network
Provides educational information for the public, patients, and healthcare professionals about the varied urologic diseases.

American Institute for Cancer Research (ACIR)
1759 R Street NW
Washington, DC 20069
800-843-8114 (Nutrition Hot Line)
202-328-7744 (In Washington, DC)
The AIRC is the only major national cancer organization that supports research and provides public education exclusively in the area of diet, nutrition and cancer. Offers free publications.

American Lung Association
1740 Broadway
New York, NY 10019-4374
212-315-8700
To conquer lung disease and promote lung health.

Biological Therapy Institute Foundation
P.O. Box 681700
Franklin, TN 37068
615-790-7535
A leading resource for physician and patient information regarding the use of biopharmaceuticals in cancer therapy.

Bone Marrow Transplant (BMT) Newsletter
1985 Spruce Avenue
Highland Park, IL 60035
708-831-1913
Publishes bi-monthly newsletter and a book on issues of concerns to patients. Provides attorney referrals for those having difficulty obtaining reimbursement for their treatment.

Burger King Cancer Caring Center
4117 Liberty Avenue
Pittsburgh, PA 15224
412-622-1212
Dedicated to helping people diagnosed with cancer, their families and friends cope with the emotional impact of cancer. The Cancer Caring Center is now handling calls for the Cancer Guidance Hotline.

Cancer Care Inc.
1180 Avenue of the Americas
New York, NY 10036
212-302-2400
Offers professional social work counseling and guidance to help patients and families cope with the emotional and psychological consequences of cancer.

Cancer Conquerors Foundation
P.O. Box 238
Hershey, PA 17033
800-238-6479 or
717-533-6124
Offers cancer survival training programs and self-study materials with specific emphasis on body/mind spirit integration.

Cancer Research Institute
681 Fifth Avenue
New York, NY 10022
212-688-7515 or
800-99CANCER
Supports leading-edge research aimed at developing new methods of diagnosing, treating and preventing cancer.

CAN ACT (Cancer Patients Action Alliance)
26 College Place
Brooklyn, NY 11201
718-522-4607
Provides advocacy and public policy, but does not provide services for individuals.

Cancer Support Network
Essex House, Suite L10
Baum Blvd. at S. Negley Ave.
Pittsburgh, PA 15206
412-361-8600
Provides emotional and psychological support through peer support groups, educational programs, community workshops, advocacy, and social gatherings.

Cancervive
6500 Wilshire Blvd., Suite 500
Los Angeles, CA 90048
310-203-9232
Assists cancer survivors to face, and overcome the challenges of "Life After Cancer."

Candlelighters Childhood Cancer Foundation
7910 Woodmont Avenue, Suite 460
Bethesda, MD 20814
301-657-8401
800-366-2223
Provides information, support and advocacy to families of children with cancer, and professionals who work with them.

ChemoCare
231 North Avenue West
Westfield, NJ 07090
800-55-CHEMO
908-233-1103
Offers personal one-to-one emotional support to cancer patients and their families undergoing chemotherapy and/or radiation treatment from trained and certified volunteers who have survived the treatment themselves.

Childrens Oncology Camps of America
c/o Linda Wells
7 Richland Memorial Park, Suite 203
Columbia, SC 29203
803-434-3533
Provides normal life experiences for children, their siblings, and their families.

Choice in Dying
200 Varrick Street, 10th Floor, Rm1001
New York, NY 10014
800-989-WILL
Advocates the recognition and protection of individual rights at the end of life. Provides counseling for individuals regarding preparing and using advance directives and durable powers of attorney for healthcare.

Coping **Magazine**
2019 North Carothers
Franklin, TN 37064
615-790-2400
Fax 615-791-4719
A bi-monthly publication which is the only nationally-distributed consumer magazine for people whose lives have been touched by cancer.

Corporate Angel Network (CAN)
Westchester County Airport Bldg. 1
White Plaines, NY 10604
914-328-1313
*Helps cancer patients bridge the miles between home and needed treat-
ment using corporate aircraft.*

Encore Plus
YWCA of the U.S.A.
624 9th St., NW 3rd Floor
Washington, D.C. 20001
202-628-3636
*Post-operative program for women that consists of peer support and
exercise.*

Families Against Cancer (FACT)
P.O. Box 588
Dewitt, N.Y. 13214
315-466-5326
*Advocacy agency that provides information to the public that justifies
increasing federal dollars to research cancer for early diagnosis and
intervention and provides educational materials on cancer prevention and intervention.*

Friends Network
P.O. Box 4545
Santa Barbara, CA 93140
805-565-7031
*A national non-profit organization which offers the only national color
cancer activities newslette –* The Funletter *— which benefits children
with cancer.*

International Myeloma Foundation
2120 Stanley Hills Drive
Los Angeles, CA 90046
800-452-CURE
Promotes education for physicians and patients about myeloma, its treatment and management. Funds research, holds clinicaland scientific conferences. Publishes a quarterly newsletter – Myeloma Today.

Susan G. Komen Breast Cancer Foundation
5005 LBJ Freeway, Suite 370
Dallas, TX 75244
800-462-9273
Their mission is to eradicate breast cancer as a life threatening disease by advancing research, education, screening and treatment.

Leukemia Society of America
600 Third Avenue
New York, NY 10016
800-955-4LSA (educational materials)
212-573-8484 (general information)
Dedicated to seeking the cause and eventual cure of leukemia and related cancers. Nationwide programs include; research, patient aid, public and professional education. The Society offers local family support group programs, free of charge, open to patients, family and friends.

Lymphoma Research Foundation of America, Inc.
2318 Prosser Avenue
Los Angeles, CA 90064
310-470-4912
A research organization that also provides a support system for lymphoma patients across the country.

Make Today Count
c/o Connie Zimmerman
Mid-America Cancer Center
1235 E. Cherokee
Springfield, MO 65804
800-432-2273
A mutual support organization that brings together persons affected by a life-threatening illness so they may help each other.

National Alliance of Breast Cancer Organizations (NABCO)
9 E. 37th Street, 10th floor
New York, NY 10016
212-719-0154
Source of information on breast cancer. Advocates for legislative and regulatory concerns of breast cancer community.

National Bone Marrow Transplant Link (BMT Link)
29209 Northwestern Hwy., Suite 624
Southfield, MI 48034
800-LINK-BMT
Reduces the burdens of those affected by bone marrow transplantation and promotes public understanding and peer support.

National Brain Tumor Foundation
785 Market Street, Suite 1600
San Francisco, CA 94103
800-934-CURE
Pursues two major goals; providing support and education for brain tumor patients, and finding a cure through research.

National Breast Cancer Coalition
1707 L Street NW, Suite 1060
Washington, DC 20036
202-296-7477
A grassroots advocacy movement of more than 300 member organizations and thousands of individuals working through a National Action Network, dedicated to the eradication of breast cancer through action, policy and advocacy.

National Cancer Institute (NCI)
Cancer Information Service
Building 31, Room 10A16
9000 Rockville Pike
Bethesda, MD 20892
800-4-CANCER
Provides a nationwide telephone service for cancer patient and their families and friends, the public, and health care professionals that answers questions and sends booklets about cancer.

National Cancer Survivors Day (NCSD) Foundation
2019 North Carothers, Suite 100
Franklin, TN 37064
615-794-3006
NCSD is America's nationwide, annual celebration of life for cancer survivor's their families, friends and oncology teams. NCSD is celebrated on the first Sunday in June of each year in communities throughout America.

National Coalition for Cancer Research (NCCR)
426 C Street NE
Washington, DC 20002
202-544-1880
Educates the public and elected officials about the need to provide a supportive environment for the successful implementation of the National Cancer Act.

National Coalition for Cancer Survivorship (NCCS)
1010 Wayne Avenue, 5th floor
Silver Spring, MD 20910
301-650-8868
Exists to enhance the quality of life for cancer survivors and to promote an understanding of cancer survivorship.

National Hospice organization (NHO)
1901 N. Moore Street, Suite 901
Arlington, VA 22209
800-658-8898
A resource for hospice professionals, volunteers and the general public for terminally ill patients and their families.

National Kidney Cancer Association
1234 Sherman Avenue, Suite 200
Evanston, IL 60202
708-332-1051
Works to increase the survival of kidney cancer patients and improve their care by providing information, sponsoring research and acting as an advocate on behalf of patients.

National Lymphedema Network
2211 Post Street, Suite 404
San Francisco, CA 94115
800-541-3259
Disseminates information on the prevention and management of primary and secondary lymphedema to the general public as well as health care professionals.

National Marrow Donor Program
3433 Broadway Street NE, Suite 400
Minneapolis, MN 55413
800-MARROW-2
A congressionally authorized network which maintains a computer-ized data bank of available tissue-typed marrow donor volunteers nationwide.

Oley Foundation
214 Hun Memorial
Albany Medical Center A-23
Albany, NY 12208
800-776-OLEY
Support for home parenteral and/or enteral nutrition therapy con-sumers and their families through a newsletter, conferences, meetings, outreach and support activities.

PDQ (Physician Data Query)
800-4-CANCER
PDQ is the National Cancer Institute's computerized listing of up-to-date and accurate information for patients and health professionals on the latest types of cancer treatments, research studies, clinical trials, new and promising cancer treatments, and organizations and doctors involved in caring for people with cancer. To access PDQ, doctors may use an office computer or the services of a medical library. Doctors and patients can also get information by calling the number above.

Patients Advocates for Advanced Cancer Treatments (PAACT)
1143 Parmelee NW
Grand Rapids, MI 49504
616-453-1477
An association for both patients and physicians for diagnostic and therapeutic treatments of prostate cancer.

R.A. Bloch Cancer Foundation, Inc.
The Cancer Hotline
4410 Main Street
Kansas City, MO 64111
816-932-8453
Helps people diagnosed with cancer have the best possibility of beating it as easily through informational resources, peer counseling, medical second opinions and support groups.

Ronald McDonald House
One Kroc Drive
Oak Brook, IL 60521
708-575-7418
Offers a refuge from the hospital, a "home-away-from-home."

Support for People with Oral and Head and Neck Cancer, Inc. (SPOHNC)
P.O. Box 53
Locust Valley, NY 11560
516-759-5333
Self-help program of support. Addresses the broad emotional, psychological and humanistic needs of these cancer survivors, empowering each to take an active role in his or her recovery.

The Chemotherapy Foundation
183 Madison Avenue, Suite 403
New York, NY 10016
212-213-9292
Supports laboratory and clinical research to develop more effective methods of diagnosis and therapy for the control and cure of cancer. Conducts professional and public education programs and provides free patient/public information booklets.

The Skin Cancer Foundation
245 5th Avenue, Suite 2402
New York, NY 10016
212-725-5176
Provides public and medical education programs, and support for medical training and research. Helps reduce incidence, morbidity, and mortality of skin cancer.

The Wellness Community
2716 Ocean Park Blvd., Suite 1040
Santa Monica, CA 90405
310-314-2555
Provides free psychosocial support to people fighting to recover from cancer, as an adjunct to conventional medical treatment. 14 facilities nationwide.

United Ostomy Association, Inc.
36 Executive Park, Suite 120
Irvine, CA 92714
800-826-0826
714-660-8624
Association of ostomy chapters dedicated to complete rehabilitation of al ostomates.

US TOO International, Inc.
930 North York Road, Suite 50
Hinsdale, IL 60521
800-808-7866
708-323-1002
Provides prostate cancer survivors and their families emotional and educational support through an international network of chapters.

Y-ME National Breast Cancer Organization
212 West Van Buren, 4th floor
Chicago, IL 60607
800-221-2141
312-986-8228 (24-hour hotline)
Hotline counseling, educational programs, and self-help meetings for breast cancer patients, their families and friends.

Y-ME Men's Support Line
M–F 9am–5pm CST
Men can call the Y-ME 800 number and request to speak to a male counselor. The counselor most closely matched in experience to the caller will return the call within 24 hours.

Editor's Note: *The above listing represents organizations that operate on a national level. There are many excellent local organizations too numerous to list. To locate them, call your local cancer treatment center, or local American Cancer Society office.*

Reprinted by permission of *Coping* Magazine

Financial Assistance — Where to Look

Although cancer can cause extensive financial damage to many families, there is help out there. Many organizations offer financial assistance in the form of monetary gifts, free or reduced-cost services and products. However during the emotional roller coaster of diagnosis and treatment, cancer survivors and their families have little time to search for these sources of aid. The editors of *Coping* magazine have compiled the following list to make "getting help" a little easier.

Cancer Fund of America

CFA is a Delaware Corporation which provides or assists in the provision of such items as oxygen, chemotherapy, transportation, medications, dressings, bed pads, diapers, nutritional dietary supplements, mastectomy, ostomy, and laryngectomy supplies. Special request for funds are also available.

147

For more information on the types of financial assistance CFA offers, write to 2901 Breezewood Lane, Knoxville, TN 37921, or call (615) 938-5281.

Directory of Pharmaceutical Manufacturers' Indigent Patient Programs

The directory is available from the Special Committee on Aging, United States Senate, chaired by Senator David Pryor of Arkansas. It contains information about drugs which are used for a variety of illnesses and may not be an extensive resource. To obtain a copy of this directory call (800) PMA-INFO.

The American Cancer Society (ACS)

The ACS offers a wide variety of free services and support groups. However, availability may vary from community to community. Some chapters of the ACS may offer temporary housing for patients during cancer related treatment or checkups. Others may provide loan or gift items such as supplies, equipment, dressings, wigs and turbans. ACS volunteers may assist cancer survivors in obtaining transportation to and from treatment facilities. Limited financial assistance may also be available for some cancer survivors. Contact your local American Cancer Society, listed in your telephone book.

The Hill-Burton Program

The Federal Government also administers the Hill-Burton program, through which many medical facilities and hospitals provide free or low-cost care. Hill-Burton hospitals receive construction and modernization funds from the government and are required by law to provide some services to people who cannot afford to pay. For more information about eligibility and to obtain a list of Hill Burton hospitals in your area, you may call (800) 638-0742, or for Maryland residents (800) 492- 0359.

The Leukemia Society of America

The Leukemia Society of America offers a variety of aid for patients with leukemia, the lymphomas and multiple myeloma. Financial assistance is limited to expenditures not covered by other sources such as third party insurers, government assistance, etc., and as determined by the patient aid committee.

Drugs, x-ray therapy, blood transfusion and transportation may be covered by some of the existing financial aid programs of the Leukemia Society or the Director of Service Programs at the National Office (212) 573-8484.

Y-ME

In addition to the free educational and support services offered through Y-ME local chapters, the organization hosts a wig and prosthesis bank. A selection of donated wigs and prostheses is available for women with limited financial resources.

Write to 212 W. Van Buren Street, Chicago, IL 60607, or call the hotline at (800) 221-2141.

Many pharmaceutical companies offer indigent programs for cancer survivors where drugs are provided free of charge or at a reduced cost. Patients are highly encouraged to ask their healthcare providers to contact the companies that manufacture the drugs they are taking. In most cases, applications must be made by a physician.

In addition to these programs, many local support and government organizations may provide financial assistance to the medically needy. Discuss your financial needs with your hospital social worker, healthcare provider and patient accounts representative to investigate all possible means of assistance.

Reprinted by permission of *Coping* Magazine.

Glossary

absorption — taking up of substances by the body tissues

analgesic — a drug that can relieve pain without loss of consciousness

anemia — a condition in which the concentration of hemoglobin in the blood is below the normal for the age and sex of the patient

anthropometric measurements — comparative measurements taken to reflect fat reserves and nutritional status of the body

arginine — an amino acid that helps reduce blood ammonium levels

astheni — loss of strength; weakness

anorexia — lack or loss of appetite

antibiotics — drugs that can destroy or interfere with the development of infections, bacteria, and other living organisms invading the body

antibody — part of the body's defense formed in response to an antigen

cachexia — severe malnutrition, weakness, and muscle wasting resulting from a chronic disease

calorie to nitrogen ratio — a formula used to calculate the number of calories needs to spare protein

catheter — a hollow flexible tube placed into a vessel through which to inject or withdraw fluids

chemotherapy — treatment or prevention of disease by means of chemical substances

clinical — pertaining to the direct care of patients

complete blood count (CBC) — a count of the number of blood cells, both red and white, and platelets

depression — emotional state characterized by despair, discouragement, and feelings of sadness

digestive tract — the organs and glands of the system that food passes through to be broken down and absorbed

edema — swelling of any part of the body due to a collection of fluid in the intercellular spaces of tissues

endoscope — an instrument used by the physician to examine organs or a cavity, so they may be removed or tissue samples taken; in placing a gastrostomy tube this is the instrument that is used to examine the stomach area

Glossary

endoscopy — any diagnostic test performed with an endoscope

enteral — taken into the body through the alimentary canal

fiber — any substance of plant origin which is undigested by human alimentary tract enzymes; fiber is often referred to a bulk or roughage

gastroenterologist — a physician that specializes in diseases of the digestive tract, including the stomach, intestines, gallbladder, and bile ducts

gastrointestinal (GI) — relating to the stomach and intestines

gastrostomy — a connection forming a pathway directly into the stomach

hematocrit — the volume percentage of red blood cells of whole blood

hemoglobin — the oxygen-bearing portion of red blood cells

hormone — a chemical secretion produced by an organ or part of the body and carried in the bloodstream to another organ or part to stimulate or retard its function; produced by endocrine glands and in the gastrointestinal tract

hyperalimentation — the intravenous administration of large amounts of nutrients for therapeutic purposes

immune response — the body's response of forming antibodies or activating lymphocytes to destroy foreign substances in the body

153

immunity — the physiologic state which makes the body able to recognize materials as foreign to itself and to neutralize, eliminate, or metabolize them without injury to its own tissue

infusion — the introduction of fluids into a vessel

infusion pump — a device that regulates specific amounts of fluid to be delivered to a patient

internal radiation — implantation of a radioactive substance directly into tissue needing radiotherapy

jejunostomy — the formation of a permanent opening through the abdominal wall into the jejunal part of the small intestines

kwashiorkor — protein malnutrition

marasmus — protein-calorie malnutrition

metastasis — transfer of a disease from its primary site to a distant location

NG — Nasogastric

negative nitrogen balance — protein intake is less than protein loss

nitrogen balance — an equilibrium of protein in the body

oncologist — a physician specializing in the treatment of cancer

oncology — the scientific study of tumors

parenteral — taken into the body in a way other than through the alimentary canal

platelet — a disk shaped body in the bloodstream that aids in the clotting of blood

positive nitrogen balance — protein intake is higher than protein loss

protein — the major building component of muscles, blood, skin, hair, and nails

radiation therapy — treatment or prevention of disease by means of high energy rays

red blood cells — the cells that transport oxygen to the tissues and remove carbon dioxide; a reduced number of red blood cells can be the cause of anemia

side effects — certain reactions to drugs or radiation patients can have as a result of treatment

total parenteral nutrition — an aggressive feeding method to provide all necessary nutrient to patients unable to eat or eat enough, whose GI tract may not be functioning; this is administered through a catheter into the superior vena cava

tumor — an overgrowth of tissue

vein — a vessel that carried blood toward the heart or one on the heart wall which returns blood to the right atrium

vitamins — compounds essential in small quantities for normal metabolic processes of the body

white blood cells — blood cells that are responsible for fighting infection; there are actually several types of white blood cells

white blood count — The number of white blood cells per cubic centimeter

X-ray — high speed gamma rays used to take pictures of the inside of the body for diagnostic purposes

Bibliography and Recommended Reading

Adibi, D.A.; Fogel, M.R.; Agrawal, R.M.: "Comparison of free amino acids and dipeptide absorption in the jejunum of sprue patients." *Gastroenterology* 67: 586-591, 1974.

Adibi, S.A.: "Intestinal transport of dipeptides in man: Relative importance of hydrolysis and intact absorption." *J. Clin. Invest.* 50:2266-2275, 1971.

Adibi, S.A.; Soleimanpour, M.R.: "Functional characterization of dipeptide transport system in human jejunum." *J. Clin. Invest.* 53:1368-1373, 1974.

Adibi, S.A.; Mercer, D.W.: "Protein digestion in human intestines as reflected in luminal, mucosal and plasma amino acid concentration after meals." *J. Clin. Invest.* 52:1586, 1973.

Adibi, S.A.: "Metabolism of branch chained amino acids in altered nutrition." *Metabolism* 15:1287-1302, 1976.

Allwood, M.C.: "Compatibility and Stability of TPN Mixtures in Big Bags." *J. Clin. Hosp. Pharm.* 9(3):181-198, Sept. 1984.

American Dietetic Association: "Position of the American Dietetic Association: Cost Effectiveness of Medical Nutrition Therapy," *ADA Reports,* Volume 95, Number 1, Jan. 1995.

American Society for Parenteral and Enteral Nutrition: Reported by Nathene Stark, R.D., "Keynote address 13th Clinical Congress News," Feb. 5–8, 1989.

Ames, B.N.: "Dietary carcinogens and anticarcinogens: oxygen radicals and degenerative diseases." *Science,* 221:1256-1260, 1983.

Anderson, C.E.: Energy and metabolism; in Schneider, H.A.; Anderson, C.E.; Coursin, D.B. (eds): *Nutritional Support of Medical Practice,* ed2. New York: Harper & Row Publishers Inc., 1983, pp10-22.

Angelillo, V.A.; Sukjdarshan, B.; Durfee, D.; et al: "Effects of low and high carbohydrate feedings in ambulatory patients with chronic obstructive pulmonary disease and chronic hypercapnia." *Ann. Intern. Med.* 103: 883-885, 1985.

Arnold, C.: "Nutrition intervention in the terminally ill cancer patient." *J. Am. Dietetic Assoc.* 86:522-523, 1986.

Askanazi, J.; Nordenstrom, J.; Rosenbaum, S.H.; et al: "Nutrition for the patient with respiratory failure: Glucose vs. fat." *Anesthesiology* 54:373-377, 1981.

Askanazi, J.; Elwyn, D.H.; Silverberg, P.A.; et al: "Respiratory distress secondary to a high carbohydrate load: A case report." *Surgery* 87: 596-598, 1981.

Askanazi, J.; Weissman, C.; Rosenbaum, S.H.; et al: "Nutrition and the respiratory system." *Crit. Care Med.* 10:163-172, 1982.

Baker, D.J.: "10 Years of TPN at Home." *Am. J. Nurs.* 4(10):1248-1249, Oct. 1984.

Barbul, A.; Rettura, G.; Levenson, S.M.; Seifter, E.: "Arginine: A thymotropic and wound-healing promoting agent." *Surgical Forum*, XVIII:101-103, Oct. 1977.

Barrocas, A.; Jastram, C.; Romain, C.: "The bridle: Increasing the use of nasogastric feedings." *Nutr. Supp. Serv.* 2(8):8-10, 1982.

Barroso, A.O.; Diener, J.R.: "Nutritional Assessment: An Important Prognostic Tool in Surgical Patients." *JPEN 2*, Abst. 6 (1978):201.

Bayless, T.M.: "Recognition of lactose intolerance." *Hosp. Pract.*, Oct. 1976, pp 97-102.

Bastian, C.; Driscoll, R.: "Enteral tube feeding at home," in Rombeau, J.; Caldwell, M. (eds): *Enteral and Tube feedings.* Philadelphia: W.B. Saunders Co., 1984, pp 494-512.

Bell, S.J.; Coffey, L.M.; Blackburn, G.L.: "Use of total parenteral nutrition in cancer patients." *Top. Clin. Nutr.* 1:37-49, 1986.

Bernard, M.A.; Jacobs, D.O.; Rombeau, J.L.: *Hospitalized Patients.* Philadelphia, W.B. Saunders, 1986.

Bistrian, B.R.; Blackburn, G.L.; et al. "Protein Status of General Surgical Patients." *JAMA* 230:858-860, 1974.

Bistrian, B.R.; Blackburn, G.L.; et al. "Prevalence of Malnutrition in General Medical Patients." *JAMA* 235:1,567-1,570, 1976.

Bistrian, B.R.; Blackburn; G.L.; Scrimshaw, N.S.; et al: "Cellular immunity in semi-starved states in hospitalized adults." *Am. J. Clin. Nutr.,* 28:1148-1155, 1975.

Bistrian, C.; Driscoll, R: "Enteral Tube Feeding in the Home" in Rombeau, J.; Caldwell, M. (eds): *Enteral and Tube Feeding.* Philadelphia: WB Saunders Co., 1984, pp494-512.

Bivens, B.A.; Hyde, G.L.; Schatello, C.R.; et al: "Physiopathology and Management of Hyperosmolar Hyperglycemic Nonketotic Dehydration." *Surg. Gynecol* 154:534- 540, 1982.

Black, M.L.; Galucci, B.B.; Katakkas, S.B.: "The nutritional assessment of patients receiving cancer chemotherapy." *Oncol. Nurs. Forum* 10:53-58, 1983.

Blackburn, G.L.; Flatt, J.P.; Hensle, T.W.: "Peripheral amino acid infusions." (In) *Total Parenteral Nutrition.* Fischer, J.E. (ed). Boston, Little, Brown Co., 363-394, 1976.

Blackburn, G.L.; Reinhoff, H.; Miller, J.D.B.; Bistrian, B.R.; Flatt, J.P.; Maini, B.S.: "Amino acid infusion after surgical injury." (In) *Current Concepts In Parenteral Nutrition.* Gree, J.M.; Soeters, P.B.; Wesdorp, R.I.; Phaf, C.W.; Fischer, J.E.; (ed). The Hague, Martinus Nijhoff Medical Division, 299-311, 1977.

Blackburn, G.L.; Maini, B.S.; Bistrian, B.R.; et al: "Surgical Nutrition" in Halpern, S.L. (ed): *Quick Reference to Clinical Nutrition.* Philadelphia, J.P. Lippincott Company, 1979.

160

Blackburn, G.L.; Bristrian, B.R.: "Nutritional care of the injured and/or septic patient." *Surg. Clin. North Am.* 56:1195-1224, 1976.

Blackburn, G.L.; Bristrian, B.R.; Maini, B.S.; et al: *Manual for nutritional/metabolic assessment of the hospitalized patient.* Presented at the 62nd Annual Clinical Congress of the American College of Surgeons, Chicago, Oct. 11–15, 1976.

Block, A.S.: "Special Needs of the Home Enteral Patient." *Nutr. Supp. Serv.* 3(9): 8-9,13-14, 1983.

Bond, J.H.; Levitt, M.D.: "Factors Affecting the Concentration of Combustible Gases in the Colon During Colonoscopy." *Gastroenterology,* 1975; 68:1445-1448.

Bouletreau, P.; Delafosse B.; Auboyer, C.; Motin, J: "Branch chained amino acids in cirrhotic encephalopathy." *J. Parent. Enteral Nutr.* 3:(4):289, 1979 (Abstract #4).

Bozzetti, R.;Pagnoni, A.M.; Del Vecchio, M.: "Excessive caloric expenditure as a cause of malnutrition in patients with cancer." *Surg. Gynecol. Obstet.,* 1980: 150; 229-234.

Bozzetti, F.: "Is Enteral Nutrition a Primary Therapy in Cancer Patients?" *Gut* (England): 35 (1 suppl) pS 65-8, Jan. 1994.

Braverman, E.R.; Pfeiffer, C.C.: *The Healing Nutrients Within,* New Canaan, Conn., Keats Publishing, 1987.

Brennan, M.F.; Burt, M.E.: "Nitrogen metabolism in cancer patients." *Cancer Treat. Rep.,* 1981: 65 (suppl 5); 67-78.

Brennan, M.F.: "Total Parenteral Nutrition in the Cancer Patient." *N. Engl. J. Med.,* 1981: 305: 375-382.

161

Broviac, J.W.; Scribner, B.H.: "Prolonged Parenteral Nutrition in the Home." *Surg. Gynecol. Obstet.* 139:24-28, 1974.

Brown, S.E.; Light, R.W.: "What is now known about protein-energy depletion: When COPD patients are malnourished." *J. Respir. Dis.* May 1983, pp36-50.

Bruner, L.; Suddarth, D: *The Lippincott Manual of Nursing Practice.* Philadelphia: J.B. Lippincott, 1974.

Burkoff, M.; Carlson, S.; Cleland, B.; et al: *Nutrition Guidance for the Cancer Patient.* University of Iowa, Iowa City, 1981.

Burt, M.E.; Stein, T.P.; Schade, J.G.; et al: "Effect of total parenteral nutrition on protein metabolism in man," abstracted. *Am. J. Clin. Nutr.* 1981: 34:628.

Buse, M.G.; Reidd, S.S.: "Leucine. A possible regulator of protein turnover in muscle." *J. Clin. Invest.* 56:1250-1261, 1975.

Buss, C.L: "Nutritional support of cancer patients. *Primary Care* 14:317-329, 1987.

Butterworth, C.: "The Skeleton in the Hospital Closet." *Nutrition Today.* March/April 1974.

Buzby, G.P.; Mullen, J.L.; Stein, T.P.; et al. "Host-Tumor interaction and nutrient supply." *Cancer.* 1980: 45;2940-2948.

Buzby, G.P.; Steinberg, J.J.: "Nutrition in cancer patients." *Surg. Clin. N. Am.* 61:691-700, 1981.

Cahill, G.E.: "Starvation in Man." *New England Journal of Medicine.* 282, mo. 12 (1970): 668-675.

Calloway, D.H.: "Dietary components that yield energy." *Environ. Biol. Med.* 1:175-186, 1971.

Cerra, F.B.; Upson, D.; Angelico, R.; et al: "Branched chains support postoperative protein synthesis." *Surg.* 92: 192-199, 1982.

Cerrullo, T.C.: "The Legal Considerations of Implementing a TPN Program." *U.S. Pharmacist.* 4:21, 1979.

Chasseaud, L.F.: "The role of glutathione and glutathione S-transferases in the metabolism of chemical carcinogens and other electrophilic agents." *Advances in Cancer Research.* 29:176-244, 1975.

Chaudhari, A.; Dultta, S.: "Alterations in tissue glutathione and angiotensin converting enzyme due to inhalation of diesel engine exhaust." *J. Toxicol. Environ. Health.* 9(2):327-337, 1982.

Chencharick, J.D.; Mossman, K.L.: "Nutritional consequences of the radiotherapy of head and neck cancer." *Cancer.* 51:811-815, 1983.

Clague, M.B.; Keir, M.J.; Wright, P.D.; Johnston, IDA: "The importance of nutrition in the postoperative period." *J. Parent. Enteral Nutr.* 3(4):311, Abstract #136, 1979.

Cohn, S.H.; Gartenhaus, W.; Sawitsky, A.; et al: "Compartmental body composition of cancer patient by measurement of total body nitrogen, potassium and water." *Metabolism.* 1981:30;222-229.

Cook, G.C.: "Independent jejunal mechanisms for glycine and glycyglycine transfer in man in vivo." *Br. J. Nutr.* 30:13-19, 1973.

Copeland, E.M. III; MacFadyen, B.V.; Lanzotti, V.J.; et al. "Intravenous hyperalimentation as an adjunct to cancer chemotherapy." *Am. J. Surg.* 1975; 129:167-173.

Copeland, E.M. III; Daly, J.M.; Dudrick, S.J.: "Nutrition and cancer." *Int. Adv. Oncol.* 4:1-13, 1981.

Copeland, E.M.; MacFadyen, B.V. Jr.; Souchon, E.A.; et al: "Intravenous Hyperalimentation and Cancer." University of Texas Medical Schools at Houston.

Costa G.; Donaldson, S.: "The nutritional effects of cancer and its therapy." *Nutr. Cancer.* 1980; 2:22-29.

Coulston, A.M.; Darbininian, J.A.: "Nutrition management of patients with cancer." *Top. Clin. Nutr.* 1:26-36, 1986.

Covelli, H.D.; Black, J.W.; Olsen, M.S.; Beekman, J.F.: "Respiratory failure precipitated by high carbohydrate loads." *Ann. Intern Med.* 95:579-581, 1980.

Craft, I.L.; Geddes, D.; Hyde, C.W.; Wise, I.J.; Mathews, D.M.: "Absorption and malabsorption of glycine peptides in man." *Gut.* 9:425-437, 1986.

Crosley, M.A.: "Watch out for the nutritional complications of cancer." *RN.* 48:22-27, 1985.

Cuthbertson, D.; Zagreb H: "The metabolic response to injury and its nutritional implications." *JPEN.* 3:108-129, 1979.

Daly, J.M.; Copeland, E.M.; Dudrick, S.J.: "Effects of Intravenous Nutrition on Tumor Growth and Host Immunocompetence in Malnourished Animals." *Surgery.* 84:655-658. Nov. 1978.

Darling vs. Charleston. Community Memorial Hospital. 50 ILL. App. 2d 253, 200 N.E. 2d 149,189, 1964.

Desai, S.P.; Bistrian, B.R.; Moldawer, L.L.; et al: "Plasma amino acid concentrations during branched chain amino acid infusions in stressed patients." *J. Trauma.* 22:747-752, 1982.

DeWys, W.D.: "Pathophysiology of cancer cachexia: Current understanding and areas for future research." *Cancer Res.* 42 (suppl): 721S-726S, 1982.

DeWys, W.D.; Begg, C.; Lavin, P.T.; et al: "Prognostic effect of weight loss prior to chemotherapy in cancer patients." *Am. J. Med.* 1980: 69:491-497.

Dickerson, J.W.T.: "Nutrition and the patient with cancer." *Proc. Nutr. Soc.* 40:31-35, 1981.

Dickerson, J.W.T.: "Nutrition in the cancer patient: A review." *JR Soc. Med.* 77:309-315, 1984.

Dudrick, S.J.; Wilmore, D.W.; Vars, H.M.; et al: "Long-term TPN with Growth, Development, and Positive Nitrogen Balance." *Surgery* 64: 134-142, 1968.

Dudrick, S.J.; Jensen, T.G.; Rowlands, B.J.: "Nutritional Support: Assessment and Indications." in Dietel (ed): *Nutrition in Clinical Surgery.*

Elwyn, D.H.; Weissman, C: "Respiratory effects of nutrients in depleted patients," in Winters, R.W.; Greene, H.L. (eds): *Nutritional Support of the Seriously Ill Patients.* New York: Academic Press, 1983, 223-229.

Ericksson, S.; Hagenfeldt, L.; Wahren, J.: "Influence of branched chain amino acids on arterial amino acid levels: Key role of Leucine." *J. Parent. Enteral Nutr.* 3(4):290, 1979 (Abstract #7).

Ericksson, S.; Hagenfeldt, L.; Wahren, J.: "A comparison of the effects of intravenous infusion of individual branched chain amino acids on blood amino acid levels in man." *Clin. Sci.* (England) 60/1:95-100, 1981.

Fairclough, P.D.; Silk, D.B.A.; Webb, J.P.W.; Clark, M.L.; Dawson, A.M.: "A reappraisal of 'osmotic' evidence of intact peptide transport." *Clin. Sci. Mol. Med.* 53:241, 1977.

Fairclough, P.D.: "Jejunal absorption of water and electrolytes in man. The effect of amino acids, peptides, and saccharides." MD thesis, University of London, 1978.

Falke, R.M.: "Nutritional therapy in advanced cancer." *Postgrad. Med.* 78:83-90, 1985.

Felig, P.: "Amino acid metabolism in man." *Ann Rev. Biochem.* 44:933-955, 1975.

Fogel, M.R.; Ravitch, M.M.; Adibi, S.A.: "Absorptive and digestive function of the jejunum after jejunoileal bypass for treatment of human obesity." *Gastroenterology* 71: 729-733, 1976.

Food and Nutrition Board, National Research Council: "Recommended Dietary Allowances," ed 9. Washington, DC: *National Academy of Sciences,* 1980.

Forman, H.J.; Rotman, E.I.; Fisher, A.B.: "Roles of selenium and sulfur-containing amino acids in protection against oxygen toxicity." *Lab. Invest.* 49(2):148, 1983.

Francois, G.; et al: "Branched amino acids. Role and value in parenteral nutrition." *Ann. Anesthesiol. Fr.* 21:71-74, No. 1, 1980.

Freund, H.R.; Ryan, J.A.; Fischer, J.E.: "Amino acid derangements in patients with sepsis: Treatment with branched chain amino acid rich infusions." *Ann. Surg.* 188(1):423-430, 1978. See also *J. Parent. Enteral Nutr.* 2(3):Abstract #63, 1978.

Freund, H.R.; James, H.H.; Fischer, J.E.: "Nitrogen sparing mechanisms of singly administered branched chain amino acids in the injured rat." *Surgery.* 90:237-243. No. 2, 1981.

Freund, H.; Yoshimura, N.; Lunetta, L.; Fischer, J.E.: "The role of the branched chain amino acids in decreasing muscle catabolism in vivo." *Surgery.* 83:611-618, 1978. See also *J. Parent. Enteral Nutr.* 2(3):Abstract #48, 1978.

Freund, H.; Hoover, H.C. Jr.; Atamiam, S.; Fischer, J.E.: "Infusion of the branched chain amino acids in postoperative patients. Anticatabolic properties." *Ann. Surg.* 190(1):18-23, 1979.

Freund. H.; Fischer, J.E.: "The branched chain amino acids: valine, leucine and isoleucine alone are sufficient for short term inhibition of postoperative muscle catabolism." *J. Parent. Enteral Nutr.* 3(4):289, Abstract #5, 1979.

167

Friedman, M.; Gumbmann, M.R.: "The utilization and safety of isometric sulfur-containing amino acids in mice." *J. Nutr.*, 114:2301-2310, 1984.

Fujii, S.; Dale, G.L.; Beutler, E.: "Glutathione-dependent protection against oxidative damage of the human red cell membrane." *Blood*, 63(5):1096-1101, 1984.

Gallagher-Alfred, C.: "Nutrition Suggestions for Meeting the Needs of Terminally Ill Patients." Columbus, Ohio. Riverside Methodist Hospital.

Garfinkel, F.; Robinson, S.; Price, C.: "Replacing carbohydrate calories with fat calories in enteral feeding for patients with impaired respiratory function." ASPEN 9th Clinical Congress Abstracts. *JPEN* 9:106, 1985.

Gershwin, M.E.; Beach. R.S.; Hurley, L.S.: (1983): "Trace metals, aging and immunity." *J. Immunol Geriatr.*, Soc. 31, 374.

Goodwin, W.J. Jr: "Nutritional Management of the Head and Neck Cancer Patient." *Med. Clin. North Am.*, 77 (3)p 597-610, May 1993.

Gormican, A.; Liddy, E.: "Nasogastric tube feedings : Practical considerations in prescription and evaluation." *Postgrad. Med.* 53:71-76, 1973.

Grant, A.: "Nutritional Assessment Guidelines." Seattle, Wash: Cutter Laboratories, 1979. aud FA, Becker, D.S.; Finkelstein, G.: "Unreceived Meals Source of Malnourishment." *Hospitals.* Feb. 1982. 47-48.

Grant, J.P.; Curtas, M.S.; Kelvin, F.M.: "Flouroscopic placement of nasojejunal feedings tubes with immediate feeding using a nonelemental diet." *JPEN* 7:299-303, 1983.

Grant, M.M.: "Nutritional interventions: Increasing oral intake." *Sem. Oncol. Nurs.* 2:36-43.

Grant, A.; DeHoog, S.: "Nutritional Assessment and support." ed 3. Seattle, Wash., 1985.

Green, G.M.: "Cigarette smoke: protection of alveolar macrophages by glutathione and cystine." *Science,* 162:810-811, 1968.

Griggs, B.A.; Hoppe, M.C.: "Update: Nasogastric tube feeding." *Am. J. Nurs.* 79:481-485, 1979.

Gutwein, I.; Baer, J.; Holt, P.R.: "The Effect of a Formula Diet on Preparation of the Colon for Barium Enema examination: Impact on Health Care and Cost." *Arch. Intern. Med.* 141: 993-996, 1981.

Habior, A.; Danowski, S.T.: "Effect of D-penicillamine on liver glutathione." *Res. Commun. Chem. Pathol. Pharmacol.* 34(1):153-156.

Hanson, R.L.: "Predictive criteria for length of nasogastric tube insertion for tube feeding." *JPEN* 3:160-163, 1979.

Harris, B.A.; Probert, J.C.: "Nutrition and metabolism in cancer patient: A review." *NZ Med. J.* 9 4;227-229, 1981.

Harvey, J.: "Feeding for therapy." *Nurs. Mirror.* 160;32-34, 1985.

Heatley, R.V.; Williams, R.H.P.; Lewis, M.H.: "Postoperative intravenous feeding-a controlled trial." *Postgrad Med. J.* 1979; 55:541-545.

Hecker, A.L.; Kies, C.; Butler, R.J.; et al: "Nutritional adequacy and gastrointestinal tolerance of a peptide-based elemental diet, crystalline amino acid diets and other defined formula diets." *Aktuelle Ernahrungsmedizin in Klinik und Praxis* 5:95-99,1980.

Heys, S.D.: "Nutrition and Malignant Disease: Implications for Surgical Practice." *Br. J. Surg.* 79 (7)p 614-23, July 1992.

Ho, C.S.; Gray, R.R.; Goldfinger, M.; et al: "Percutaneous gastrostomy for enteral feeding." *Radiology.* 156:349-351, 1985.

Holman, R.T.: "Essential fatty acid deficiency, in Progress in the Chemistry of fats and Other Lipids." Oxford: Pergamon Press 9:275-348, 1968.

Holroyde, C.P.; Gabuzda, T.G.; Putnam, R.C.; et al: "Altered glucose metabolism in metastatic carcinoma." *Cancer Res.* 1975: 35:3710-3714.

Holmes, S.: "Dietary problems in the cancer patient." *Nurs. Mirror.* 157:27-30.

Holt, P.R.: "Medium chain triglycerides: A useful adjunct in nutritional therapy." *Gastroenterology.* 53:961-966, 1967.

Harvey, C.C.; Duncan, G.D.; Wilson, W.C.: "Effects of limited tocopherol intake in man with relationships to erythocyte hemolysis and lipid oxidations." *Am. J. Clin. Nutr.* 4:408-419, 1956.

Hoppe, M.C.: "Nutritional Support in the Home." *Hospital Material Management Quarterly.* Vol. 7, No. 3, 1986.

Howard, L.: "Home Parenteral and Enteral Nutrition in Cancer Patients." *Cancer.* 72 (11 suppl) pp3531-41, Dec. 1993.

Hsu, J.M.: "Lead toxicity as related to glutathione metabolism." *J. of Nutr.* III:26-33, 1981.

Husain, S.; Dunlevey, D.: "Possible role of glutathione (GSH) in phencyclidine (PCP) toxicity and its protection by N-acetylcysteine (NAC)." *The Pharmacologist.* 243(3): 1982.

Iapichino, G.; Radrizzani, D.; Solca, M.; et al: "Influence of Total Parenteral Nutrition on Protein Metabolism Following Acute Injury: Assessment by Urinary 3-Methylhistidine Excretion and Nitrogen Balance." *JPEN* 9(1): 42-46, Jan.–Feb. 1985.

Irwin, M.M.: "Enteral and parenteral nutrition support." *Sem. Oncol. Nurs.* 2:44-54, 1986.

Issell, B.F.; Valdivieso, M.; Zaren, H.A.; et al: "Protection against chemotherapy toxicity by IV hyperalimentation." *Cancer Treat Rep.* 62:1139-1143, 1981.

Janes, E.M.H.: "The importance of follow up in the nutritional care of the cancer patient." *Acta. Chir. Scand.* 5079 SUPPL): 162-166, 1981.

Jeejeebhoy, K.N.; Langer, B.; Tsallas, G.; et al: "Total Parenteral Nutrition in the Home Studies in Patients Surviving 4 Months to 5 Years." *Gastroenterology.* 71:943-953, 1976.

Jensen, G.E.; Clausen, J.: "Glutathione peroxidase activity in vitamin E and essential fatty acid-deficient rats." *Ann. Nutr. Metab.* 25:27-37.

Johndrow, P.D.: "Administer Hyperalimentation in the Home?" *Home Healthcare Nurse.* 2(5):27-31, Nov.–Dec. 1984. (S740;114)

Kaminski, M.V.: "Enteral Hyperalimentation." *Surg. Gynecol. Obstet.* 143:12-16, 1976.

Keithley, J.K.: "Proper nutritional assessment can prevent hospital malnutrition." *Nursing.* 79 9(2):68-72, 1979.

Kern, K.A.; Bower, R.H.; Atamian, S.; et al: "The effect of a new branched chain enriched amino acid solution on postoperative catabolism." *Surg.* 92:780-785, 1982.

Klipstein, F.A.; Corcino, J.J.: "Malabsorption of essential amino acids in tropical sprue." *Gastroenterology.* 68: 239-244, 1975.

Kim, J.A.; Baker, D.G.; Hahn, S.S.; Goodchild, N.T.; Constable, W.C.: "Topical use of N-acetylcysteine for reduction of skin reaction to radiation therapy." *Sem. in Oncol.* 10(1):86-88, 1983.

Kinney, J.M.: "Basic concepts of energy metabolism, in Current Approaches to Nutrition of the Hospitalized Patient." Abbott-Ross Research Conference, Amelia Island, Florida, 1975, pp 1-6.

Kinney, J.M.; Long, C.L.; Duke, J.H.: "Carbohydrate and nitrogen metabolism after injury," in Porter, R.; Knight, J.(eds): Ciba Foundation Symposium; Energy Metabolism and Trauma, 1970, pp103-126.

Kinney, J.M.: "Energy requirements of the surgical patient, in American College of Surgeons, Committee on Pre and Postoperative Care: Manual of Surgical Nutrition." Philadelphia: W.B. Saunders Co. 1975, pp223-235.

Kinney, J.M.; Gump, F.E.: "The Metabolic Response to Injury, in Pre and Post Operative Care" (Dudrick, S.J., ed).

Koretz, R.L.: "Nutritional Support: Fixing Nitrogen, Fixing Patients." *Gastroenterology* 107(2) p594-6, August 1994.

Krey, S.H.; Murray, R.L.: *Dynamics of Nutritional Support.* Norwalk, Conn. Appleton-Century-Crofts. 1986.

Kuna, P.; Petyrek, P.; Dostal, M.: "Modification of toxic radioprotective effects of cystamine by glutathione in mice." *Radiobio. Radiother.* 599-601, May 1978.

Lafleur, M.V.M.; Woldhuis, J.; Loman, H.: "Effects of sulphydryl compounds on the radiation damage in biologically active DNA." *J. Radiat. Biol.* 37(5):493-498, 1980.

Larsson, A.; Orrenius, S.; Holmgren, A.; Mannervik, B: "Functions of glutathione, biochemical, physiological, toxicological and clinical aspects." *Annal. Biochem.* 139(1):126, 1984.

Lawson, D.H.; Richmond, A.; Nixon, D.W.; et al: "Metabolic approaches to cancer cachexia." *Annu. Rev. Nutr.* 1982; 2:277-301.

Lawson, D.H.; Stockton, L.H.; Bleier, J.C.; Acosta, P.B., Heymsfield, S.B.; Nixon, D.W.: "The effect of a phenylalanine and tyrosine restricted diet on elemental balance studies and plasma aminograms of patients with disseminated malignant melanoma." *Amer. J. Clin. Nutr.* 41(1):73-84, 1985.

Leibach, F.H.; Pillion, D.J.; Mendicino, J.; Pashley, D.: "The role of glutathione in transport activity in kidney," in *Functions of Glutathione in Liver and Kidney,* eds. Sies and Wendel. New York: Springer-Verlag, 170-180, 1978.

Leone, P.L., Mequid, M.: "The Impact of Nutritional Status and Therapy on Immunity." *Contemporary Surgery 21.* Dec. 1982: 21-29.

Letsou, A.P.; Connaughton, M.C.; O'Donnell, T.P.: "Nutrition Survey of a University Hospital Population." *JPEN* 1:4, 40A, 1977.

Levitt, M.D.: "Production and Excretion of Hydrogen Gas in Man." *N. Engl. J. Med.* 1969; 281:122-217.

Levy, L.; Vredevoe, D.L.: "The effect of N-acetylcysteine on cyclophosphamide immunoregulation and antitumor activity." *Sem. in Oncol.* 10(1):7-16, 1983.

Lindmark, L.; Ekman, L.: "Metabolic effects of nutritional support to cancer patients." *Med. Oncol. Tumor Pharmacother.* 2:213-217, 1985.

Long, C.L.: "Energy and protein requirements in stress and trauma, part 2." *Crit. Care Nurs. Curr.* 2:7-12, 1984.

Long, C.L., Schaffel, W.; Geiger, J.W.; et al: "Metabolic response to injury and illness: Estimation of energy and protein needs from indirect calorimetry and nitrogen balance." *JPEN* 3: 452-456, 1979.

Lum, L.L.; Gallagher-Allred, C.R.: "Nutrition and the cancer patient: A cooperative effort by nursing and dietetics to overcome problems." *Cancer Nurs.* 7:469-474, 1984.

Lundholm, K.; Bylund, A.C.; Schersten, T.: "Glucose tolerance in relation to skeletal muscle enzyme activities in cancer patients." *Scan. J. Clin. Invest.* 1977: 37;267-272.

Lundlum, K.; Edstrom, S.; Ekman, L.; et al: "Metabolism in peripheral tissues in cancer patients." *Cancer Treat. Rep.* 1981; 65(suppl 5):79-83.

Malloy, M.H.; Rassin, D.K.: "Cysteine supplementation of total parenteral nutrition: The effect on beagle pups." *Ped. Res.* 18(8):747-751, 1984.

"Malnutrition seen in Illinois hospitals." *American Medical News* 28, No.21 (May 24/31, 1985):22.

Margie, J.D.; Black, A.S.: *Nutrition and the Cancer Patient.* Radnor, PA. Chilton, 1983.

Martin, D.J.; Cerrullo, T.C.: "Medicolegal Considerations in Nutritional Support." *Nutritional Support Services.* 1:4,21-22. 1981.

Mathews, D.W.; Adibi, S.A.: "Peptide absorption." *Gastroenterology.* 71:151-161. 1976.

Matthews, D.M.: "Protein absorption." *J. Clin. Pathol.* 5(suppl 24):29, 1971.

Matthews, D.M.: "Intestinal absorption of peptides." *Physiol. Rev.* 55:537, 1975.

McArdle, A.; Reid, E.C.; Laplante, M.P.; Freeman, M.B.: "Prophylaxis Against Radiation Injury." *Archives Surgery.* Vol. 12. 1986.

Meguid, M.M.; Eldar, S.; Wahba, A.: "The delivery of nutritional support: A potpourri of new devices and methods." *Cancer* 55:279-289, 1985.

Miller, L.F.; Rumack, B.H.: "Clinical safety of high oral doses of acetylcysteine." *Sem. in Oncol.* 19(1):76-85, 1983.

Mills, B.J.; Lindeman, R.D.; Lang, C.A.: "Differences in blood glutathione levels of tumor-implanted or zinc-deficient rats." *Amer. Inst. Nutr.* III(9):1586-1592, 1981.

Milner, J.A.; "Stepanovich LV: Inhibitory effect if dietary arginine on growth of Ehrlich ascites tumor cells in mice." *J. Nutr.* 109:489-493, 1979.

Milner, J.A.; Garton, R.L.; Burna, R.A.: "Phenylalanine and tyrosine requirements of immature beagle dogs." *J. Nutr.* 114:2212-2216, 1984.

Morgan, L.R.; Holdiness, M.R.; Gillen, L.E.: "N-acetylcysteine: its bioavailability and interaction with ifosfamide metabolites." *Sem. in Oncol.* 10(1):56-61, 1983.

Moriarty, K.J.: "Dietary nitrogen formulation: Does it really matter?" *Gut* 225:a430, 1981.

Mullen, J.L.; Certner, M.H.; et al: "Implications of Malnutrition in the Surgical Patient." *Arch. Surg.*, 114:121-125, 1979.

Mullen, J.L.; Buzby, G.P.; Gertner, M.H.; et al: "Protein synthesis dynamics in human gastrointestinal malignancies." *Surgery.* 87:331-338, 1980.

Nasset, E.S.; Schwartz, P.; Weiss, H.V.: "The digestion of proteins in vivo." *J. Nutr.* 56zz;83, 1955.

Nehme, A.E.: "Nutritional Support of the Hospitalized Patients-the Team Concept." *JAMA* 243:1,906-1,908, 1980.

Newey, H.; Smyth D.H.: "Intracellular hydrolysis of dipeptides during intestinal absorption." *J. Physiol.* (Lond) 152:367, 1960.

Nixon, D.W.; Heymsfield, S.B.; Cohen, A.E.; et al: "Protein-calorie undernutrition in hospitalized cancer patients." *Am. J. Med.* 68:683-690, 1980.

Nixon, S.E.; Mawer, G.E.: "The digestion and absorption of proteins in man: 1. The site of absorption." *Br. J. Nutr.* 24:227, 1970.

Norton, J.A.; Stein, T.P.; Brennan, M.F.: "Whole body protein synthesis and turnover in normal man and malnourished patients with or without cancer." *Ann. Surg.* 1981; 194:194:123-128.

Norton, J.A.: "Cancer Cachexia," *Crit. Rev. Oncol. Hematol.* 7 (4) p289-327, 1987.

Novi, A. Am.; Florke, R.; Stukenkemper, M.: "The effect of glutathione (GSH) on aflatoxin B1-induced tumors." Presented at New York Academy of Science, Feb. 17, 1982.

Oliver, I.; et al: "Preventation and dissolution of cystine stones by D-penicillamine." *Harefuah*, 84(1):11-12, 1973.

Paauw, J.D.; McCamish, M.A.; Dean R.E.; Ouellette, T.R.: "Assessment of caloric needs in stressed patients." *J. Am. Coll. Nutr.* 3:51-59, 1984.

Page, C.; Clibon, U.: "A method of enterally feeding defined formula diet." *Am. J. IV Ther. Clin. Nutr.* 9:9-38, 1982.

Pareira, M.D.: "Therapeutic nutrition with tube feeding." *JAMA* 156;810-816, 1954.

Patel, M.S.; Owen, O.E.; Goldman, L.I.; et al: "Fatty acid synthesis by human adipose tissue." *Metabolism.* 24;161-173, 1975.

Pearson, D.; Shaw, S.: *Life Extension*, Warner Publishing, NY, NY, 1983.

Peters, C.; Fischer, J.E.: "Studies on nitrogen ratio for total parenteral nutrition." *Surg. Gyencol. Obstet.* 151:1-8, 1980.

Pfeiffer, C.C.: "Mental and Elemental Nutrients," New Canaan, CT: Keats Publishing, Inc., 1975.

Powell, Tuck.; Goode, A.W.: "Principles of enteral and parenteral nutrition." *Br. J. Anesth.* 53:169, 1981.

Prescott, L.F.; Park, J.; Ballantyne, A.; Adriaenssens, P.; Proudfoot, A.: "Treatment of paracetamol (acetaminophen) poisoning with N-acetylcysteine." *Lancet.* August 1977.

Ragins, H.; Shinya, H.; Wolff, W.I.: "The Explosive Potential for Colonic Gas During Colonoscopic Electrosurgical Polypectomy." *Surg. Gynecol. Obstet.* 138:554, 1974.

Reilly, J.J.: "Does Nutrition Management Benefit the Head and Neck Cancer Patient?" *Onc.* 4 (6) p105-15, 115-6, June 1990.

Robbins, G.E.; Trowbridge, F.L.: "Anthropometric techniques and their application," in Simko, M.D.; Cowell, C.; Gilbride, J.A. (eds): *Nutrition Assessment*, Rockville, Md: Aspen Publications, pp85-89, 1984.

Rothman, M.M.; Katz, A.B.: "Analysis of feces," in Bockus, H.L. (ed): *Gastroenterology*, ed 2. Philadelphia: W.B. Saunders Co., Vol. 2, pp 694-725, 1964.

Rucker, B.B.; Holmstedt, K.A.: *Home Infusion Therapy Industry*. Hambrecht, 1984.

Schneider, H.A.; Anderson, C.A.; Coursin, D.B.: (1977) *Nutritional Support of Medical Practice; Clinical and biochemical findings, Vit. E.* 120-121. Harper & Row.

Schwartz, G.F.; Green, H.L.; Bendon, M.L.; et al: "Combined parenteral hyperalimentation and chemotherapy in the treatment of disseminated tumors." *Am. J. Surg.*, 121:169-173, 1971.

Scribner, B.H.; Cole, J.J.; Christopher, T.C.: "Longterm TPN-The Concept of an Artificial Gut." *JAMA* 212:457, 1970.

Seltzer, M.H.; et al: "Instant Nutritional Assessment." *JPEN* 3: 157-159, 1979.

Seltzer, M.H.; et al: "Instant Nutritional Assessment in the Intensive Care Unit." *JPEN* 5 (1981): 70-72.

Silk, D.B.A; Perrett, D.; Clark, M.L.: "Jejunal and ileal absorption of dibasic amino acids and an arginine-containing dipeptide in cystinuria." *Gastroenterology* 68:1426, 1975.

Silk, D.B.A.: "Peptide absorption in man." *Gut.* 15:494-501, 1974.

Silk, DB.A.; Dawson, A.M.: "Intestinal absorption of carbohydrate and pr.otein in man," in Crane, R.K. (ed): *Intestinal Review of Physiology*, Baltimore: University Park Press, p151, 1971.

Smith, F.P.; Kisner, D.; Schien, P.S.: "Nutrition and Cancer: Prospects for clinical research." *Nutr. Cancer* 2:34-39, 1980.

Spencer, R.; Palmisano, D.J.: "Specialized Nutritional Support of Patients- A Hospital's Legal Duty?" *Quality Review,* Bulletin 11, No. 5 (May 1985): 160-163.

Spencer, R.; Palmisano, D.: "Nutritional Support as a Legally Recognized Standard of Patient Care."*Hospital Material Management Quarterly* 7, No.3 (1986):xx-xx.

Solassol, C.; Joyeux, H.: "Ambulatory parenteral nutrition," in Fischer, J.E. (ed): *Total Parenteral Nutrition.* Boston, Little Brown & Co. 1976, pp 285-301.

Solomons, N.W.: "The Use of H2 Breath-Analysis Breath in Gastrointestinal Diagnosis." *Curr Concepts Gastroenterology.* 1983; 8:30-40.

Steffee, W.P.: "Malnutrition in Hospitalized Patients." *JAMA* 244; 2, 630-2, 635, 1980.

Steiger, E.: "Home Parenteral Nutrition: Components, Applications, and Complication." *Postgrad. Med.* 75(b): 95-102, May 1984.

Steiger, E.J.; et al: "Standards for Nutritional Support-Home Patients." *Washington, D.C.: American Society for Parenteral and Enteral Nutrition.* 1985.

Stryer, L.: *Biochemistry,* Freeman Publishing, 1975.

Takeda, Y.; Tominaga, T.; Tei, N.; Litamura, M., Taga, S.; Murase, J.; Taguchi, T.; Miwatani, T.: "Inhibitory effect of L-arginine on growth of rat mammary tumors induced by 1,12 dimethylbenz (a) antracene." *Cancer Res.* 35:2390-2393, 1975.

Teitelman, R.: "Skeletons in the Closet." *Forbes,* April 19, 1984: 156-157.

Theologides, A.; "Nursing Care of the Cancer Patient with Nutritional Problems." *Report of the Ross Oncology Nursing Roundtable.* Columbus Ohio: Ross Laboratories, 1981, p 1-31.

Thomas, C.W.; Scholz, R.W.; Reddy, C.C.; Massaro, E.T.: "Inhibition of in vitro lipid peroxidation by reduced glutathione in rat liver microsomes." *Fed. Proc.* 41(5), 1982.

Twomey, P.L.; Patching, S.C.: "Cost-Effectiveness of Nutritional Support." *JPEN* 9, No. 1 (1985) 3-10.

Unverferth, D.V.; Mehegan, J.P.; Nelson, R.W.; Scott, C.C.; Leier, C.V.; Hamlin, R.L.: "The efficacy of N-acetylcysteine in preventing doxorubicin- induced cariomyopathy in dogs." *Sem. in Oncol.* 19(1):2-6, 1983.

Uren, J.R.; Lazarus, H.: "L-cyst(e)ine requirements of malignant cells and progress toward depletion therapy." *Cancer Treatment Reports,* 63(6):1073-1079, 1979.

Vandenbergh, E.; Van de Woestijne, K.P.; Gyselen, A.: "Weight changes in the terminal stages of chronic obstructive pulmonary disease." *Am. Rev. Respir. Dis.* 95:556-566, 1967.

Vitamin E. General Mills, 1973.

Wagner, W.H.; Silberman, H.: "Lipid-based Parenteral Nutrition and the Immunosuppression of Protein Malnutrition." *Arch. Surg.* 119(7):809-810, July 1984. (s705;161)

Warnold, I.; Lundholm, K.; Schersten, T.: "Energy balance and body composition in cancer patients." *Cancer Res.* 1978; 38:1801-1807.

Waterhouse, C.; Jeanpretre, N.; Keilson, J.: "Gluconeogenesis from alanine in patients with progressive malignant disease." *Cancer Res.* 1979; 39:1968-1972.

Weisner, R.L.: "Hospital Malnutrition-A Prospective Evaluation of General Medical Patients During the Course of Hospitalization." *American Journal of Clinical Nutrition.* 32 (Feb. 1979): 418-426.

Werlin, S.L.: "Growth Failure in Crohn's Disease: An Approach to Treatment." *JPEN* 5:250-253, 1981.

Whitney, E.N.; Cataldo, C.B.: *Understanding Normal and Clinical Nutrition.* New York: West Publishing Co., 1983.

Wilcutts, H.D.: "Nutrition Assessment of 1000 Surgical Patients in an Affluent Suburban Community Hospital." (Abstract)*JPEN* 1:4 25, 1977.

Willard, M.D.; Gidsdorf, R.B.; et al. "Protein-Calorie Malnutrition in a Community Hospital." *JAMA* 243:1,720-1,722, 1980.

Wilmore, D.W.: *The Metabolic Management of the Critically Ill.* New York: Pleum Medical Book Company, 1977.

Wright, B.; Robinson, L.: "Enteral feeding tubes as drug delivery systems." *Nutr. Supp. Serv.* 6(2):33, 1986.

Yarbro, W.; et al: (eds) "N-acetylcysteine: a significant chemo protective adjunct." Chicago; Seminars on Oncology x (1) (Suppl. 1), 1983.

Young, V.R.: "Energy metabolism and requirements in the cancer patient." *Cancer Res.* 1977; 37:2336-2347.

Yoshimura, K.; Iwauchi, Y.; Sugiyama, S.; Kuwamura, T.; Odaka, Y.; Satoh, T.; Kitagawa, H.: "Transport of L-cysteine and reduced glutatione through biological membranes." *Research Commun. in Chem. Path. and Pharm.*, 37(2):171-186, 1982.

Index

malnutrition 11, 12, 16, 27, 35,
  36, 51, 53, 68, 69, 70, 71, 72,
  79, 85, 93, 94
manganese 76
marasmus 35, 69, 71
meals on wheels 20, 23
medical nutritionals 42, 43,
  45, 95
metabolism 16, 75, 76
mouth sores 32, 33, 97

N
nausea 28, 29, 50, 65, 79, 89
nitrogen balance 72
nutritional assessment 78, 95
nutritional assessment 58, 63,
  64, 68, 69, 77, 78, 95, 96
nutritional supplements 42, 43,
  44
nutritional support teams 14

P
partial parenteral nutrition 50, 82
positive nitrogen balance 72
protein malnutrition 35, 36, 69,
  70, 71, 72
protein-calorie malnutrition 35,
  69, 71

R
radiation therapy 26, 29, 38, 63

S
somatic protein 58

T
transferrin 67, 68, 78

V
visceral protein 57, 58
vomiting 25, 28, 50, 65, 77, 79

Z
zinc 21, 26, 27, 76

About the Authors

Jane Bradley

Jane Bradley holds a B.S. degree in Medical Technology from Northwest Missouri State University and she has worked with physicians, nurses, and dietitians in the nutrition field for 18 years. She and Susan have published articles on nutrition and cancer in *Coping* magazine. Jane appeared with Richard Bloch of the Bloch Cancer Center on a television program about nutrition and cancer. Jane also has presented training classes on nutrition to college nursing schools. She is a frequent speaker at state and regional conferences.

Susan Calhoun

Susan earned a B.S. degree in Nutrition and Dietetics (the American Dietetic Association's undergraduate program) from the University of Rhode Island. She is a member of the American Society for Parenteral and Enteral Nutrition. She has 12 years of experience specializing in parenteral (intravenous) nutrition.

Much of Susan's experience has been with nutrition education in the hospital environment. She has presented numerous forums to hospital professionals, for which they received continuing education credits.

NOTES

NOTES

NOTES